Under the Knife

Under the Knife

A History of Surgery in 28 Remarkable Operations

ARNOLD VAN DE LAAR

St. Martin's Press
New York

www.stmartins.com

Photo of Jan de Doot on page 13:
Thanks to the Anatomical Museum of Leiden University Medical Center

Library of Congress Cataloging-in-Publication Data

Names: Laar, Arnold van de, author.
Title: Under the knife : a history of surgery in 28 remarkable
    operations / Arnold van de Laar.
Other titles: Onder het mes. English
Description: First U.S. edition. | New York : St. Martin's Press, 2018. |
    Translation of: Onder het mes : de beroemdste patièenten en operaties
    uit de geschiedenis van de chirurgie. | Includes bibliographical
    references and index.
Identifiers: LCCN 2018019684 | ISBN 9781250200105 (hardcover) |
    ISBN 9781250200099 (ebook)
Subjects: LCSH: Laar, Arnold van de. Onder het mes. English. |
    Surgery—History.
Classification: LCC RD19 .L33 2018 | DDC 617—dc23
LC record available at https://lccn.loc.gov/2018019684

Our books may be purchased in bulk for promotional, educational,
or business use. Please contact your local bookseller or the Macmillan
Corporate and Premium Sales Department at 1-800-221-7945,
extension 5442, or by email at MacmillanSpecialMarkets@macmillan.com.

First published in Great Britain by John Murray (Publishers),
an Hachette UK company

First U.S. Edition: October 2018

10 9 8 7 6 5 4 3 2 1

Contents

Under the Knife

Introduction

Healing by Hand: Chirurgeons and Surgeons

ONE NIGHT IN 1537, after a long day of fighting in the battle for Turin, young French army surgeon Ambroise Paré lay wide awake. He was seriously troubled. The battlefield was strewn with soldiers with wounds inflicted by arquebuses and muskets, which Paré had never dealt with before. He had read in a book that you should pour boiling oil into the wound to counteract the toxic gunpowder. So he had dripped the bubbling liquid onto the bloody flesh and it had sputtered like meat in a frying pan. But there were so many wounded that his cauldron of oil was empty halfway through his round of the battlefield. With no oil left, he had to alleviate the suffering of the wounded men with an ointment of rose oil, egg yolks and turpentine. The whole night he listened to men screaming and fighting death, thinking that it was his fault. He was astounded to discover the following morning that it was the soldiers he had treated with boiling oil that had been screaming and not the others. He never used boiling oil again and would later become a great surgeon. This was a first step towards modern surgery.

Surgery must have evolved quite naturally since, as long as humans have walked the earth, they have suffered from ailments that had to be healed 'by hand'. The healer who used his hands was known as a chirurgeon, from the Greek *kheirourgia*, meaning hand (*kheir*) and work (*ergon*). Our modern word 'surgeon' derives from the same origin. Fighting, hunting, migrating, digging for roots, falling from trees, fleeing predators – the hard life of our ancestors exposed them to endless risk of injury. Tending to wounds is therefore not only the most basic of surgical procedures, but was probably also the first. Common sense tells us that we should rinse a dirty wound with water, apply pressure to a bleeding wound, and cover an open wound. If you see that the wound then heals, you'll do the same thing again next time. But in the Middle Ages, common sense was obscured by tradition. Rather than looking at the results of their actions, our medieval forefathers would follow what some great predecessor had written in an ancient book. So wounds were not cleaned, but seared with a branding iron or boiling oil and dressed with a dirty piece of cloth. Only after that dark age, during that sleepless night in Turin, did common sense prevail and a new form of surgery, based on experiment, begin to emerge.

But back to the beginning. When were our ancestors first inspired to treat infections like festering wounds, pustules, carbuncles or abscesses by cutting them open? Draining pus is the second basic surgical procedure. All you need is something sharp, like an acacia thorn, a flint arrowhead, a bronze dagger or a steel scalpel. This is how the knife made its way into surgery and we surgeons still have the old adage *ubi pus, ibi evacua* – Latin for 'where there is pus, evacuate it' – hanging above our beds.

The third basic procedure for surgeons is treating fractures. Fleeing from wolves, hunting mammoths, stumbling over rocks and tree roots – prehistoric life must have presented ample opportunities to break your bones. Was there anyone sensible enough back then to pull a broken bone straight, painful as that was for the victim? It was, in any case, not something everyone could do; you had to have the guts to do it and – much more importantly – the patient had to be willing to let you. Only someone with enough courage, authority and experience, and who showed enough empathy, would be able to win that trust. And you had to be good with your hands. And that was where the chirurgeon came in, the man who could heal with his hands.

Giving patients emergency treatment has remained part of the surgeon's work. Dealing with injuries and severe loss of blood, making sure patients can breathe and making them stable are still the primary tasks of surgeons in emergency departments in hospitals. This basis is clear and sound. Treating wounds, abscesses and fractures, and giving emergency treatment to someone in acute distress, results in grateful patients.

But going a step further and performing an operation is a completely different matter. You don't heal a wound, you make one. A sensible surgeon (and a sensible patient) will weigh up the risks. Does the operation usually succeed or fail? Are there alternatives? What will happen to the patient if I do nothing? What will happen to me if the operation is a failure? It is always a matter of seeking a balance between doing your best and not causing harm. And yet . . . Roman consul Marius had a surgeon remove his varicose veins. He survived and continued to rule for many years. Surgeon John Ranby thought it advisable to operate on Queen Caroline of England's umbilical hernia, causing her to die a miserable death. Yet his Roman colleague was given a severe reprimand and was not permitted to operate on Marius's other leg, while Ranby was knighted for his services to the royal court. Surgery can be an unpredictable profession.

Wounds, fractures, pus infections and operations leave scars, while diseases like colds, diarrhoea and migraine can disappear without leaving any trace. This difference is illustrated by two different words for 'getting better': we use 'heal' – to 'make whole' – to refer to operations, wounds, bruises and fractures, and 'cure' – to 'restore to health' – for diseases. Roughly speaking, a surgeon heals and a doctor cures. Surgeons have incidentally long been both doctors and surgeons, but they restrict themselves to problems treatable by surgical means, which are a minority of all the ailments a patient can suffer from. Most complaints do not require the intervention of a surgeon or an operation at all. The services provided by chirurgeons in the sixteenth century were so straight-forward and limited that they could perform them, as simple tradesmen, in a small shop. In Amsterdam, surgeons were so insignificant as a professional group that they shared a guild with three other trades – skate-makers, clog-makers and barbers.

Until well into the eighteenth century, wounds, infections and fractures constituted the lion's share of the limited range of complaints that surgeons treated. To that list could be added cutting or burning away misunderstood tumours and growths and, of course, bloodletting – the most popular surgical treatment which, however, had more to do with superstition than treatment. All in all, it was a rather simple and dull business. If I had been a surgeon at that time, I would certainly have taken much less pleasure in it than I do now.

As methods and knowledge improved with experience, the diversity of complaints that could be treated with surgery increased. Walking upright is one of the main causes of many of the typical complaints we suffer from as human beings. That first step, taken by our ancestors 4 million years ago, brought with it a series of medical conditions that account for a large number of surgical interventions. Varicose veins, groin hernias, piles, impaired blood supply to the legs (intermittent claudication), wear and tear of hip- and knee-joints (arthrosis), spinal hernias (slipped discs), heartburn and torn menisci in the knees are all caused by our walking on two legs.

Two complaints that account for a significant part of a surgeon's work these days did not pose a serious threat to human life until relatively recently. Cancer and hardening of the arteries (arterio-sclerosis) have made their way into our lives in the past couple of centuries, brought on by a lifestyle typified by a high-calorie diet and the consumption of tobacco. Furthermore, these diseases are usually contracted in later life and in the past you would simply have died before you got cancer or your arteries blocked up.

Clogs, a cap and a surgical mask

Modern surgeons change their clothes regularly. To do an operation they put on 'scrubs' – a clean light-blue or green top and trousers, white clogs and a cap. In the operating theatre they also wear a surgical mask and, when they are operating, a sterile operating jacket, called a surgical gown, over their scrubs and sterile rubber gloves. At the end of the nineteenth century, when it was discovered that germs could be spread via minuscule droplets of saliva in the air, surgeon Johann von Mikulicz from Breslau decided not only to speak as little as possible during an operation, but also to wear a mask over his mouth. Perhaps the cloth masks that gentlemen surgeons wore at the time were primarily intended to cover their beards, just as the operating caps were to cover their hair. In any case, according to Johann von Mikulicz, they rapidly became accustomed to them and, as he wrote in the *Centralblatt für Chirurgie* in 1897, it was as easy to breathe through the masks 'as a lady on the street breathing through her veil'. The AIDS epidemic also led to many surgeons wearing splash-proof glasses during their operations. These can be troublesome with a mask, as the glasses will fog up if the mask is not a tight fit around the cheeks and nose. Magnifying glasses known as loupes are used for precision surgery, sometimes together with a light on the forehead. The most unwieldy items of surgical clothing are the lead jackets worn under the surgical gown during operations involving X-rays, which are very heavy.

From the nineteenth century, people suddenly started to live longer due to a remarkable development in the Western world, which meant more for modern surgery than any great discovery or renowned surgeon you can name: people started to be more aware of hygiene. This led to a radical change in surgery. It is difficult to imagine why it took so long for hygiene and surgery to be linked together. We would be deeply shocked if we found ourselves in an operating theatre in the eighteenth century. The screaming must have been indescribable; blood would have been spattering in all directions, and the stench from searing the stump of an amputated limb would have made us retch. It would have been like something from a horror film.

Modern operating theatres are generally quiet places that smell of disinfectant. A vacuum may be used to remove blood or fluids. The only background noise is from the sleeping patient's heart-beat on the monitor and possibly the radio will be on, but the operating team can talk to each other freely. Yet the real difference between operations today and in the past is much more subtle, and is not immediately clear to an outsider. That difference is sterility, achieved by applying stringent rules that form the basis of all modern medicine.

In the surgical world, sterile means 'completely free from bacteria'. Our scrubs, gloves, surgical instruments and other equipment are all sterilised. They are placed in an autoclave – a kind of pressure cooker – for several hours, where they are subjected to steam, or are treated with gamma rays to kill all bacteria and other germs. During operations, we take almost draconian measures, creating a sterile zone around the wound where nothing or no one inside the zone can touch anything or anyone outside the zone. If you are part of the team, you are sterile – that means there is not a single bacterium on your clothes or gloves. To preserve that sterility, you have to observe a strict procedure in putting on the gown and gloves and in walking around the patient: always keep your hands above waist level, look at each other as you pass, turn around completely as you tie up your gown and never turn your back on the patient. To restrict the number of bacteria in the operating theatre even further, everyone wears a cap and a mask, the number of people present during the operation is kept to a minimum, and the door stays shut as much as possible.

All of these measures have produced very visible results. It used to be considered normal that pus would leak from a wound after an operation. Only a stupid surgeon did not know that. That is why you had to leave the wound open, so that the pus could get out easily. It was not until sterility could be assured that the customary wound infections could be prevented and wounds could be closed up immediately after the operation had been completed. Hygiene is thus not the only new element in surgery; stitching up wounds is also a relatively recent development.

What kind of people are surgeons? What on earth makes you want to cut into someone's body, even if they can't feel it? How can you sleep if a patient is fighting for their life after you have operated on them? How do you carry on if a patient has died as a result of you operating on them, even though you made no errors? Are surgeons insane, brilliant or unscrupulous, heroes or show-offs? There is a great deal of tension involved in being a surgeon. Operating is a wonderful thing, but the responsibility weighs very heavily.

When they operate, surgeons literally become part of the treatment of their patients, after all, their hands and their skills are the instruments. When that is the case, you have to be sure of yourself if problems arise. You ask yourself if they happened because of your personal contribution to the treatment, or whether the problems were caused by something else. After all, we never know how any medical complaint will turn out, no matter how good the treatment. Problems may also arise during the course of the disease itself. But, as a surgeon, you have to justify that course for yourself, more so than doctors, who do not use their own hands to influence it. You ask yourself whether you have done your best and done the right thing. Most surgeons conceal that perpetual doubt behind an air of self-confidence. That attitude has always determined the image of a surgeon as omnipotent and untouchable. Yet, even among the most self-confident of surgeons, this is only a front, to allow them to bear the responsibility and keep the latent feeling of guilt at a distance. Just get on with it, that is their motto.

Every surgeon has had patients die during or after their operations, even though they made no mistakes. You have to get over it and move on, as the next patient will be waiting to be treated. It is a little like a train driver who hits someone on the line, but couldn't do anything about it. The trains have to keep running. Patient deaths are dramatic events and some are easier to get over than others, depending on the circumstances, and the reasons for the operation. If the patient has cancer or has suffered a serious accident, you have no choice other than to operate. If it was elective surgery, an operation for which there was also a non-surgical alternative, or if the patient was a child, it is more difficult.

Naturally, your experience also makes a difference. It matters whether you have performed an operation five or five hundred times. Every procedure has a learning curve; there is a greater chance of complications the first few times you perform it, but that risk decreases as you gain more experience. Every surgeon has to go through this learning curve, there is no way of getting around that. In the seventeenth century Charles-François Félix de Tassy was by no means a novice, but he had never performed an operation to cut open an anal fistula when Louis XIV consulted him about this complaint. So he asked the king to give him six months and first performed the operation on seventy-five patients before daring to try it on the king. I wonder whether my first patients were aware of my comparative lack of experience when I was just beginning as a surgeon.

You also have to be physically capable of working for hours on end under pressure of time, mostly standing up and without fixed breaks, to work night shifts and then continue in the morning, write discharge letters, train young surgeons, lead your team, stay friendly, tell people bad news, give them hope, record everything you say and do, explain everything adequately, and yet never leave the next patient in the waiting room for too long.

Fortunately, the setbacks and the less pleasant aspects of the work are compensated for by the gratitude of patients and their families, and the great pleasure of doing surgical operations more than makes up for the hard work. Performing an operation is complex, but it is also enjoyable. Most of the things a surgeon has to do are quite basic and require skills you learn at nursery school, such as cutting, sewing and doing everything neatly. If I had never played with Lego as a child or enjoyed making things, I would never have suited being a surgeon. There is something else that makes surgery enjoyable: the detective work, finding out what is wrong with the patient. Looking for the underlying problem and discussing the best solution with your colleagues are welcome distractions.

The surgeon's job may seem magical for people who have nothing to do with surgery: the responsibility, skills and knowledge of a person who can save lives. That is why surgeons were often treated with great respect, even awe, portrayed as heroes who, in the face of adversity and appalling working conditions, tried to save their patients with their scalpels. But this image is often distorted. Surgeons were often indifferent, naive, unclean, clumsy and bent only on money or fame.

In this book, I recount some of the stories of my profession and look at a number of famous patients, renowned surgeons and extraordinary operations. That is not simple, as surgery is not only an interesting and exciting job, but is above all very technical. Surgery is concerned with the complex details of the functioning of the human body, and uses jargon that is almost incomprehensible to outsiders. Readers without a surgical background will have no idea what we mean, for example, by an 'acute abdominal aortic aneurysm', a 'sigmoid perforation' or a 'B-II resection'. Surgical concepts therefore need to be explained, so that everyone can understand the point of these stories. Consequently, they are not only about the history of surgery but also about how our bodies work and what a surgeon can do to make sure they keep working.

Some surgical terms may require further explanation. The words 'incision' and 'resection' come from the Latin and mean literally 'cut into' and 'take away'. 'Trauma' comes from Greek and means 'injury' or 'wound'. A trauma can be psychological, in the sense of suffering a trauma after a bad experience, but in surgery it means that something is physically damaged. 'Indication' means 'the reason for an operation', while a 'complication' is an undesired development or a calamity. Other terms can be found in the Glossary at the back of the book.

The various stories do not offer a complete history of surgery, but they do give an impression of what it was – and still is – about. What is surgery? What was it in the past? What happens during an operation? What do you need to perform one? How does the human body respond to being attacked by a knife, a bacterium, a cancer cell or a bullet? What are the principles of shock, cancer, infection and the healing of wounds and fractures? What can be repaired by an operation and what cannot? Why did the most common operations arise and who thought of them? Most of the chapters describe operations on famous figures and contain interesting details. Did you know, for example, that Albert Einstein lived much longer than was actually possible, Houdini gave his final performance while suffering from acute appendicitis,

Empress Sisi was stabbed at the age of sixty, John F. Kennedy and Lee Harvey Oswald were operated on by the same surgeon, or that a man from Amsterdam cut a stone out of his own bladder? Did you know that you have an electrical current passing through your body during an operation, and that surgeons did not start washing their hands before an operation until 150 years ago?

Some of the stories are especially dear to me. Jan de Doot, the man with the bladder stone, is a favourite because I live in Amsterdam myself, not far from where he operated on himself. And the story of the gluttonous popes also intrigues me, because I have a special interest in operating on people with obesity problems. Then there are the stories about the Shah of Persia, as I had the pleasure to be surgeon to his charming widow; and Peter Stuyvesant, because I worked for some years as a surgeon on the beautiful Caribbean island of St Martin; and the one about keyhole surgery, because I was present when my boss performed the first remote surgical procedure in history. Lastly, long ago, another surgeon from Amsterdam also wrote a book of observations on surgical practice. He was Nicolaes Tulp, portrayed by Rembrandt in his painting *The Anatomy Lesson of Dr Nicolaes Tulp*. He concluded his *Observationes Medicae* with a chapter about a chimpanzee. I follow in the footsteps of my fellow-Amsterdammer and also devote the last chapter to a special animal.

Nicolaes Tulp dedicated his book to his son. I dedicate mine to my children, Viktor and Kim, whom I have to abandon so often in the evenings or at weekends to work at the hospital.

Arnold van de Laar
Amsterdam, 2014

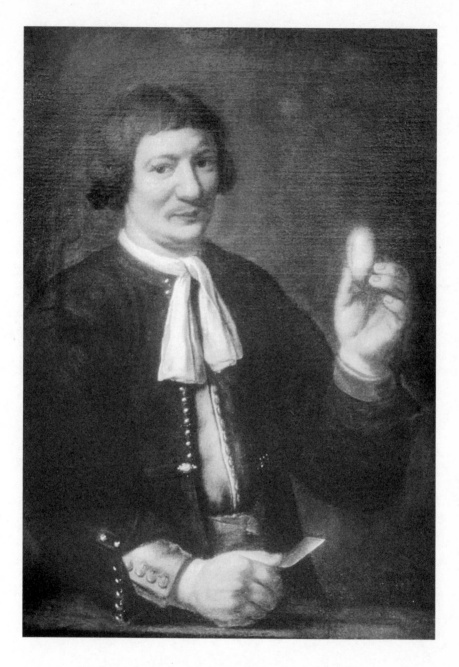

Jan Jansz. de Doot with his bladder stone and his knife,
by Carol van Savoyen, 1655.

I

Lithotomy

The Stone of Jan de Doot, Smith of Amsterdam

A EGER SIBI CALCULUM praecidens' – literally translated is 'a sick man cutting out a stone from the front himself' – is the title of a chapter in a book by Nicolaes Tulp, master surgeon and mayor of Amsterdam in the seventeenth century. Tulp describes a wide variety of disorders and other medical curiosities he encountered in his practice in the city. They include 'a twelve-day attack of hiccups', 'the mortification of a thumb after blood-letting', 'a rare cause of objectionable breath', 'a pregnant woman who ate 1,400 salted herring', 'piercing of the scrotum', 'daily urination of worms', 'pain in the anus four hours after defecation', 'pubic lice' and the rather macabre 'a hip burned off with red-hot iron'. He wrote the book *Observationes Medicae* in Latin to be read by fellow surgeons and doctors. But it was translated into Dutch without his knowledge and became a bestseller among non-medical readers. His description of the smith Jan de Doot, who had cut out his own bladder stone, must have been a favourite, as Jan was portrayed in action on the title page of the book.

Jan de Doot lost all confidence in Tulp's profession and literally took the matter into his own hands. He had suffered from the bladder stone for many years and had twice looked death in the face as a surgeon tried and failed to remove it. This operation is known as a lithotomy, literally 'stone-cutting'. In those days, the mortality rate of a lithotomy – that is, the odds that you would die from it – were 40 per cent. One of the most important attributes of a successful stone-cutter's practice was a good horse, so that he could get as far away as possible before the victim's family could call him to account. The profession of stone-cutter was therefore – like that of tooth-puller and cataract-pricker – by nature a travelling occupation. The advantage of this nomadic existence was that there were always poor wretches in the next village who were suffering so much from their ailments that they were willing to take the risk – and pay for it, too.

De Doot had twice survived the 40 per cent odds of dying under the knife – a combined risk statistically speaking of 64 per cent. So it was pure luck that he was not yet dead. The pain was excruciating, his discomfort unbearable and his nights sleepless. Bladder stones have occurred throughout human history. They have been found in ancient mummies and there have been reports of stone-cutting since time immemorial. Bladder-stone pain was an everyday complaint, like scabies and diarrhoea, and so ubiquitous that you could compare it to present-day ailments like headache, backache or irritable bowel syndrome.

Bladder stones are caused by bacteria and are a direct result of a lack of hygiene. It is a misconception that urine is by nature dirty. In normal circumstances, the yellow fluid is completely free of any kind of pathogens from its origin in the kidneys to its discharge through the urethra. Bacteria in the urine are therefore not normal. They cause blood and pus in the bladder, which can create a gritty sediment. You don't feel it at all, as long as it is still small enough to discharge in the urine. But if you have a succession of bladder infections one after the other, the sediment may become so large that it can no longer find its way out. Then it forms a stone. And, once a stone has formed in your bladder that is too big to be discharged, that tends to generate new infections. So once you had one, you could never get rid of it and, with each infection, it would get bigger. Bladder stones therefore have a characteristically layered structure, like an onion.

Why did people in the seventeenth century get bladder stones so easily, while today they are very rare? Houses in cities like Amsterdam were cold, damp and draughty. The wind blew through the cracks in the doors and window frames, the walls were wet from rising damp, and the snow came in under the front door. There was little to be done about it, so people always wore thick clothing, day and night. Rembrandt's portraits show people in fur coats wearing hats. In those days people were not able to take a daily bath in clean water. The water in the canals was sewer water. Dead rats floated in it, people defecated in it and threw their waste into it, and tanners, brewers and painters discharged their waste chemicals in it. The canals in the Jordaan district of the city were little more than extensions of the muddy ditches that passed through the surrounding pasturelands, so that cow manure flowed slowly into the River Amstel. You couldn't take a decent bath in the waters of the river, or wash out your underwear, and toilet paper had not yet been invented.

Consequently, the groins and private parts of these thickly clothed people were always dirty. The urethra, the tube for discharging urine from the body, presented only a small obstacle to bacteria entering the bladder. The best remedy from this external assault was to urinate as much as possible to rinse the urethra and the bladder clean. But that meant drinking a lot and clean drinking water was hard to come by. The water from the pump was not always trustworthy. The best way to ensure it was safe was to make soup from it. Wine, vinegar and beer could also be kept much longer and, around 1600, the average Dutch citizen would drink more than a litre of beer a day. As this did not apply to children, bladder infections often started during childhood, giving the stones plenty of time to grow.

Hippocrates and the stone-cutter

When they take the Hippocratic oath, young doctors swear by the gods to promise a number of things. They boil down to four basic principles: the duty of care (to always do your best for all those who are sick), professional ethics (respect and loyalty to colleagues), professional secrecy (privacy and discretion) and the all-embracing starting point of 'first do no harm' (*Primum non nocere* in Latin). According to Hippocrates, stone-cutting did not fulfil these requirements. In his oath, he urges doctors to leave the cutting of stones to others. Today, this specific passage is interpreted as an appeal to refer patients to a specialist if you cannot treat them yourself, but that is actually nonsense. Hippocrates meant exactly what he said and firmly placed stone-cutters outside the boundaries of medicine, with tooth-pullers, fortune-tellers, poison-mixers and other charlatans. In his time, there was probably good reason for this. No matter how much a bladder stone could make your life a misery, the chances of dying from having it cut out were probably quite high. Since then the risks of operations have been reduced a hundredfold. The fear of surgery is no longer justified, not even in the case of health problems not life-threatening. Hippocrates could only have dreamed of a time when surgical operations not only saved but also improved the quality of lives.

Any bladder infection will give three unpleasant complaints: pollakisuria (abnormally frequent urination), dysuria (pain when urinating), and urgency (a compelling urge to urinate). Since Tulp described Jan de Doot's deed as an unprecedented tour de force, Jan's bladder must have been causing him terrible pain to make him cut himself open. What complaints, in addition to those of a normal bladder infection, did the smith suffer to drive him to such desperation?

At the exit to the bladder, at the bottom of the urethra, there is a kind of pressure sensor. The sensor is stimulated when you have a full bladder, so that you feel the need to urinate. But a stone lying on the bottom of your bladder will give you the same urge, whether your bladder is full or not. And if you then try to urinate, the pressure will cause the stone to block the exit from the bladder, so that almost nothing comes out. Furthermore, the stone will press even harder against the sensor, increasing the urge. That will cause more pressure, less urine to come out, and a greater urge to urinate – enough to drive you crazy. We know that the Roman emperor Tiberius ordered his torturers to tie up their victims' penises, which of course led to such complaints. If you suffered in this way day and night, whether your bladder was full or empty, what did you care about a 40 per cent chance of survival?

For anyone who has never had a bladder stone, it must be difficult to imagine where you would need to make an incision to get the thing out. But because a stone closing off the exit from the bladder is pushed downward by the pressure, a sufferer like Jan de Doot would know exactly where it could be reached: between the anus and the scrotum. This area is called the perineum. But anyone who is familiar with the human body would never start cutting it open down there – there are too many blood vessels and sphincters in close proximity. It would be easier to access the bladder from above but that is, in turn, dangerously close to the abdomen and the intestines. Because stone-cutters were not anatomists, but crafty conmen with little understanding of what they were doing, they cut into the body from below and went straight for the stone, taking little account of the damage they could be causing to the functioning of the bladder. Most victims who survived the stone-cutter's work became incontinent.

In Jan de Doot's time, there were two ways to remove a bladder stone: the 'minor' operation (using the 'apparatus minor') and the 'major' operation (using the 'apparatus major'). The first method was described in the first century AD by the Roman Aulus Cornelius Celsus, but had already been applied for many centuries. The principle of the 'minor' operation is simple. The patient lies on his back with both legs in the air, a position still called the lithotomy position. The stone-cutter then sticks his index finger into the patient's anus. This enables you to feel the stone in the bladder in the front, through the rectum. You then pull it towards you with your finger, in the direction of the perineum. You ask the patient – or someone else – to hold the scrotum up, while you make an incision between the scrotum and the anus until you can get at the stone. Then you get the patient to press it out like a woman pushing out a baby. Someone can help him by pressing on his abdomen, or the stone-cutter can pull it out with a hook. If that all works, you then have to stop the patient from bleeding to death by applying considerable pressure to the wound for as long as possible.

It was an operation that could only be performed on men and then only up to the age of about forty. Around that age, a gland swells up that gets in the way of the incision. For that reason, the gland was called the prostate, based on the Latin *pro-status*, meaning 'standing in front of'.

The 'major' operation was described in 1522 by Marianus Sanctus Barolitanus, a new method devised by his master Joannes de Romanis of Cremona. Instead of bringing the stone to the instrument, the instruments were brought to the stone. The 'Marian operation' required the use of a large number of instruments, hence the term 'apparatus major'. The sight of all these metal tools was often enough to make the patient faint or change his mind. The 'major' operation was also conducted in the lithotomic position, but the scrotum did not need to be lifted out of the way. A bent rod was inserted into the bladder through the penis. A scalpel was used to make a vertical incision in the direction of the rod, between the penis and the scrotum, along the centre line of the perineum. A 'gorget', a grooved instrument, was then inserted into the bladder, through which the stone could be crushed and removed in fragments, using spreaders, forceps and hooks. The advantage of the 'major' operation was that the wound was actually smaller, reducing the risk of incontinence.

De Doot did not have access to all these complicated instruments, so had no choice other than to keep it simple. He only had a knife and performed the 'minor' operation by making a large, crossways incision. The smith had made the knife himself and before getting down to work – not unimportantly – had concocted an excuse to send his wife (who suspected nothing) to the fish market. The only other person present during the operation, on 5 April 1651, was his apprentice, who held his scrotum up out of the way. Tulp writes *'scroto suspenso a fratre uti calculo fermato a sua sinistra* (the brother held the scrotum up so that the stone was held in place with his left hand). From his pidgin Latin, however, it is difficult to determine which of the two men had their left index finger in Jan's rectum. Perhaps Jan tried to do everything himself and his assistant simply observed the 'operation' with growing amazement. Jan made three cuts, but the wound was still not wide enough. So he stuck both his index fingers (one of which was obviously his left one) into the wound and tore it open wider. He probably did not suffer a lot of pain and loss of blood, as he went through the scar tissue resulting from the operations he had undergone when he was younger. By pressing vigorously and, according to Dr Tulp, more by luck than judgement, the stone finally emerged, with a lot of crunching and cracking, and fell on the ground. It was larger than a chicken's egg and weighed four ounces. The stone was immortalised in an engraving, along with Jan's knife, in Tulp's book. The drawing clearly shows a longitudinal groove in the stone, probably caused by the knife.

The wound was enormous and eventually had to be treated by a surgeon, and continued to fester for many years. Carel van Savoyen's portrait of Jan, painted four years after his heroic act, shows the smith standing (not sitting!) with a bitter smile on his face and holding both stone and knife.

Not long after Jan de Doot's act of desperation, the primitive incision in the centre of the perineum would be replaced by other methods. Unfortunately, these were not without risk. In the year Jan cut the stone out of his own bladder, a man called Jacques Beaulieu was born in France. Under the name Frère Jacques, Beaulieu travelled around Europe performing the 'major' operation through an incision from the side a few centimetres off the midline. In the early years of the eighteenth century he made a name for himself performing the operation in Amsterdam. As fatalities and complications after the operation decreased, the incision became smaller and the stone could be extracted with greater precision. In 1719, John Douglas performed the first *sectio alta*, the 'high section' through the lower abdomen. This access route had always been taboo because of a warning by Hippocrates, who believed that a wound on the upper side of the bladder would always be fatal. But he was proved wrong. In the nineteenth century, lithotomy was rendered almost completely obsolete by transurethral lithotripsy, a difficult term for pulverising (-tripsy) the stone (litho) via (trans) the urethra. Narrow, collapsible forceps and files are inserted into the bladder through the penis, and used to break the stone into small fragments. In 1879, the cystoscope was invented in Vienna; this is a small visual probe that can be inserted directly into the bladder through the urethra, making it much easier to pulverise and remove stones. Prevention, however, remains the best treatment. The discovery of daily clean underwear has meant more in combating this great tormentor of mankind that any new operating method. As a consequence, genuine lithotomies are rarely performed now, and never via the perineum. Furthermore, the operation is no longer the domain of the surgeon, but the urologist.

For anyone who is still curious about how a lithotomy between the legs must have felt, the French composer Marin Marais set the 'major' operation he had himself endured in 1725 to music. The piece, for viola da gamba in E minor, is called 'Tableau de l'opération de la taille'. It lasts three minutes and describes the operation's fourteen stages from the perspective of the patient: the sight of the instruments, the fear, bracing oneself and approaching the operating table, climbing onto the table, climbing off again, reconsidering the operation, allowing yourself to be tied to the table, the incision, the introduction of the forceps, the extraction of the stone, almost losing your voice, the blood flowing, being released from the table and taken to bed.

Jan de Doot became famous throughout the country. Many people will have declared him insane. The month after the operation, he described his actions in a deed drawn up by notary Pieter de Bary in Amsterdam on 31 May 1651. It noted that 'Jan de Doot, resident in the *Engelsche Steeg*, of 30 years of age . . .' had also produced a poem about it '. . . written, rhymed and composed with his own hand'. The proud smith alluded to the fact that, although both his action and his last name suggested that he should have been dead, he was still alive:

> What wonders the whole land
> About this fortunate hand?
> Although it is a deed of man
> It's guided by God's own plan.
> When to survive was quite remote
> He gave life again to de Doot.

What must his wife have thought when she returned from the market?

2

Asphyxia

The Tracheotomy of the Century: President Kennedy

IT IS EARLY Friday afternoon at Parkland Memorial Hospital in Dallas. A forty-five-year-old man is brought into the emergency room with a gaping bullet wound to the head. Blood and brain tissue are dripping from the hole. Other patients are quickly diverted away from the department. A large number of people, all of them agitated, come in with the victim. Journalists mill around outside. The man's wife walks alongside the stretcher, her face spattered with his blood. The victim is wheeled into the trauma room and the doors close behind him. He is alone with a doctor and a nurse, while his wife waits outside in the corridor.

The doctor is twenty-eight-year-old Charles Carrico, a second-year surgical resident on duty in the Emergency Room. He recognises the victim at once. Lying in front of him, covered in blood and with a large hole in his head, is President John F. Kennedy. He is unconscious and his body is making slow, spasmodic movements. Carrico can see the president is having trouble breathing and immediately inserts a breathing tube into the windpipe through his mouth. Using a laryngoscope, a hook-shaped instrument with a small light, he looks deep into the oral cavity, pushing the tongue to one side and opening the throat as far as possible until he can see the epiglottis, the cartilaginous valve covering the entrance of the windpipe. Behind it, he can just about see the vocal cords, and he manages to squeeze the plastic tube in between them. The president's other wounds all

24

require attention, but first air has to get into his lungs. Blood is flowing slowly from a small wound in the middle of his neck. The door opens, there is a lot of commotion in the corridor. Dr Malcolm Perry, the surgeon on duty, enters the room.

As the whole world knows, Kennedy did not survive and died there in the trauma room. That same evening, far away in the Bethesda Naval Hospital in Washington DC, military pathologist Dr James Humes conducted an autopsy on the president's body, which had been flown there in all haste. Humes was aware that this was the autopsy of the century. He could not afford to make mistakes and there were plenty of people watching his every move. Men in dark suits whose identities were a mystery. In front of him lay not just a dead body. It was also the most important piece of evidence in establishing exactly what had happened that day – and that was a matter of national interest. If all the bullet wounds Humes found came from the same direction, the shooting could be the work of one man, a solo action by a disturbed lunatic. But if he were to discover that the shots came from different directions, it had to have been a coordinated attack by more than one gunman.

But Humes had a problem right from the start. No bullets showed up on the X-rays, meaning that they must have all passed through the body, each leaving an entry and an exit wound. And yet he found only three bullet wounds. Two were clearly in a straight line, a small hole in the back of the head and a larger one on the right side. The third was a small wound on the right side of the back, just below the base of the neck. As it was so small, it could have been an entry wound. Entry wounds are always smaller than exit wounds, but an exit wound from a high-velocity bullet can also be that small. Either way, the question remained where the corresponding exit or entry wound was. There was no sign of it anywhere on the body.

Kennedy was succeeded by his vice-president, Lyndon Baines

Johnson. LBJ was sworn in as president the same day in the same presidential aircraft in which Kennedy's body had been flown from Dallas to Washington. One of President Johnson's first decisions, taken exactly a week after Kennedy's death, was to set up a presidential commission chaired by Chief Justice Earl Warren, to investigate the shooting. The Warren Commission also questioned the doctors who attended Kennedy. The commission's final report is accessible to the public and the transcriptions of the doctors' testimonies can be found easily on the Internet. The following can be deduced from their accounts.

Within eight minutes of being shot in Dallas, John F. Kennedy was taken to the Emergency Room at Parkland Memorial Hospital, where he was attended by nurse Margaret Henchcliffe and surgical resident Charles James Carrico. Carrico immediately inserted a breathing tube and connected it to a respiratory machine. At that moment, thirty-four-year-old Dr Malcolm Oliver Perry entered the room. Like Carrico, he saw that the president was choking. He looked at the small wound in the middle of the front of the neck, from which blood was flowing slowly. He must have had only a fraction of a second to assess the situation and make a decision.

The president was unconscious, but his chest was rising and falling slowly. These were not normal breathing movements, however, despite the breathing tube. Either the tube was not in the right position or something else was wrong, perhaps a pneumothorax (a collapsed lung) or a haematothorax (where blood fills the chest cavity). And then there was the small wound in the front of the neck. Was it an injury to the windpipe? If Carrico's breathing tube was in the windpipe, why were there no air bubbles escaping through the wound? And what if the tube was in the wrong place, in the oesophagus (gullet) and not in the windpipe at all? That called for immediate action.

Perry took a scalpel and performed a tracheotomy – literally a cut (-*tomy*) in the neck and into the windpipe (*trachea*) to get air into the lungs. A special tracheostomy tube can then be inserted in the windpipe. Because the small bullet wound in the neck was precisely in the spot where he needed to make the incision – in the middle of the neck, just below the Adam's apple – Perry decided to use the hole for the tracheotomy, widening it horizontally on both sides with the scalpel. And that is why Hume could not find the fourth bullet hole.

After Perry, Trauma Room 1 quickly filled up with a lot of other doctors. The first two to arrive after him, Charles Baxter and Robert McClelland, immediately assisted him with the tracheotomy. While they inserted the tracheostomy tube in the windpipe, the next two doctors on the scene, a surgical resident and a urologist, placed a chest tube on either side. This is a plastic tube inserted through the chest wall, between the ribs, and into the chest cavity to drain air or blood from around the lungs in the case of a pneumothorax or haematothorax. An anaesthetist attended to the respiratory machine, heart activity was monitored by an electrocardiograph and veins were cut open in the arms to administer blood and fluid. The blood was O-negative and the fluid was lactated Ringer's solution, a solution of water and minerals.

Neurosurgeon William Kemp Clark inspected the brain injury. Because he happened to be standing there, he was also asked to remove the breathing tube from the mouth, so that Perry could replace it with the tracheostomy tube in the windpipe. As he removed the tube, Clark saw blood in the throat. A nasogastric tube was also inserted through the oesophagus into the stomach. Despite all these efforts, however, the president's breathing did not improve. He had also lost an enormous quantity of blood from the head wound, to which a nurse was applying pressure with a gauze. The doctors saw blood and brain tissue on the floor and the stretcher. After the attempts to free the airway, they could no longer feel a pulse. Clark and Perry immediately started heart massage, but this caused more blood to flow from the head wound. Dr Clark finally had the courage to stop the resuscitation and pronounced the president dead at 1 p.m., 22 minutes after he had been admitted.

Shortly afterwards the body of the president was commandeered by secret service agents and taken to the military hospital in Washington. There was no exchange of information between the doctors in Dallas and the military doctors. This led to a controversy about the bullet wounds that gave rise to many persistent and long-lasting conspiracy theories. Perry and ten other doctors in Trauma Room 1 in Dallas had not had the time to turn the president over and examine him from behind, and therefore never saw the wound in his back just below the neck and the wound in the back of his head. Immediately after the tragic events of that afternoon, Perry found himself overwhelmed by reporters at an improvised press conference. He referred to the bullet wound in the neck as an entry wound, leading the media to assume, in the first hours and days after the assassination, that there had been one or more shots from the front. This was, of course, completely at odds with the reason given for arresting Lee Harvey Oswald. The young man had been apprehended less than an hour and a half after the attack and was immediately identified as the sole gunman, even though he had shot from a position *behind* the president.

The reports on the president's death were therefore inconsistent with the autopsy report and there was a feeling that there had been a cover-up. Humes had not called Perry until the following morning and then heard about the bullet hole in the windpipe. That information was the final piece in the puzzle, as far as he was concerned: the bullet wound in the back just below the neck, a bruise on the top of the right lung that he had found in the president's chest cavity, and the hole in Perry's tracheotomy, were

The ABC of emergency medical assistance

The alphabet provides us with a useful memory aid for medical assistance in emergencies. ABC tells us the sequence of actions that need to be carried out to stabilise a patient in a life-threatening situation. A stands for airway: this has to be free, or the patient will choke to death within minutes. That usually entails inserting a breathing tube through the mouth and between the vocal cords into the windpipe. This is known as intubation. If it does not work for some reason, the windpipe has to be cut open immediately through the front of the neck. This is called a tracheotomy. There is no time to hesitate, as every second counts. 'When you think of tracheotomy, perform it!' This is how urgent and life-saving it can be. B stands for breathing: you have to make sure the patient's lungs are getting enough oxygen and expelling sufficient carbon dioxide. This can be ensured by connecting the patient to a respiratory machine. Insufficient gas exchange between the blood and the external environment causes the brain, the heart and all other vital organs to not receive enough oxygen, creating a risk that they will stop functioning. This is known as ischaemia. The muscles can do without oxygen for six hours, but the brain only four minutes. Secondly, the pH level of the blood falls if the carbon dioxide it contains is not exhaled. Acidic blood damages the organs even more and has a detrimental impact on the circulation. That is what the C stands for. You have to stabilise the circulation, make sure the patient does not bleed to death, and keep the heart and blood pressure under control. And then there is a D and an E . . .

exactly in line, and were consistent with a shot from behind, just like the wound in the head. That meant the president had been killed by two shots from behind. One assassin, no coup. And yet, many people continued to attach more importance to the spontaneous account of the heroic young surgeon, who had seen the wounds with his own eyes while the president was still alive, than to the report of a secret autopsy conducted in the middle of the night at a military hospital.

The explanation of Kennedy's bullet wounds is to be found on an amateur film shot by Abraham Zapruder who, thanks to his secretary, made a crystal-clear recording of the motorcade – and therefore the attack on the president – in clear focus. Zapruder had stood on a wall to get a better view and, since he had vertigo, his secretary had held on to his legs while he was filming. The recording, not released until fifteen years later, shows the images that are now so familiar to everyone, of fragments of the president's head flying through the air and of his desperate wife Jackie climbing over the boot of the moving car. Less well known is what the film shows five seconds before the shot to the head. It is hardly noticeable but, suddenly, Kennedy grimaces and grabs his throat with both hands. No one seems to notice and, while everyone is smiling and waving cheerfully, the president seems to be choking.

This is what happened. The horrific head wound was caused by the third shot. The second shot hit Kennedy in the back and passed diagonally through his windpipe, below his vocal cords. That prevented him from calling out or screaming and no one noticed that he was suffocating. The bullet exited the front of his neck and hit Texas governor John Connally, who was sitting in front of Kennedy, in the chest, the right wrist and the left thigh. Because of its seemingly bizarre trajectory, this bullet was to become known as the 'magic bullet', aka Warren Commission Exhibit Number 399. A reconstruction based on the Zapruder film shows, however, that the trajectory of the bullet was not at all as bizarre as it seemed. Before this second shot, a first shot was fired. But it missed its target and wounded a spectator, James Tague, on his right cheek. The noise of the first shot caused

Connally to turn around in the car and pick up his Stetson, so that all the wounds he and Kennedy suffered as a result of the second shot were in a line. This line can even be retraced to the open window on the sixth floor of the Texas School Book Depository. Whether it was Lee Harvey Oswald who had been at the window or another shooter remains unclear, as Oswald denied the killing and was shot dead himself two days later.

What actually happened, in medical terms? The two bullet wounds threatened the life of the president in three different ways. The shot to the head had blown away a large part of the right half of his brain. We will never know how much exactly and which part: John F. Kennedy's brain has gone missing. But no matter how horrific a wound to the brain may be, it is not always fatal. Damage to the right half of the brain causes paralysis (hemiplegia), reduced sensitivity (hemihypoesthesia) or a deficit in attention to stimuli (hemineglect) on the left side of the body, or decreased vision in the left side of the visual field (hemian-opsia). It can also cause personality change (frontal lobe disorder), an inability to perform simple mathematical tasks (acalculia), the loss of appreciation for music (amusia) and loss of memory (amnesia). But the capacity to speak and understand language is largely located in the left half of the brain, while the most impor-tant zones for regulating respiration and consciousness are further away, in the brain stem. There would therefore not have been much left of Kennedy as a person, but his body could probably have lived on with the results of his brain injuries.

Nor was the serious loss of blood from his head necessarily lethal. Severe blood loss can be replenished with fluid and blood transfusions, as long as the heart can maintain the blood pressure. Kennedy must have had sufficient blood pressure when he arrived at the hospital, because his pulse was still detectable and he was still moving. The autopsy revealed no other unexpected internal bleeding. But it is difficult, of course, to say after the fact whether it would have been possible to stem the bleeding from the gaping wound in the brain.

A much more immediate threat was the wound to the windpipe. In the eight minutes between the shot through his windpipe and Carrico inserting the breathing tube, Kennedy had been unable to breathe. Insufficient oxygen in the blood for too long is known as asphyxia, the medical term for suffocation. It quite quickly causes damage to the brain and the brain stem as – of all the parts of the body – they survive the shortest time without oxygen. Initially, the damage is reversible; the victim loses consciousness and faints. Then the damage becomes irreversible. The victim can no longer regain consciousness, but still breathes independently. That is what we call a coma. Finally, the damage becomes fatal and the systems for maintaining life, the regulation centres for our consciousness, respiration and blood pressure in the brain stem, shut down completely. The damage to the respiration centre in the brain stem resulting from a lack of oxygen was what caused the strange movements the president made as he suffocated. The autopsy revealed no collapsed lungs or large quantities of blood in and around the lungs. Inserting a breathing tube or conducting a tracheotomy could therefore perhaps have saved his life, if only they had been performed earlier. Today, unconscious victims are never moved without a breathing tube being inserted first. The tube is put in place by the ambulance crew, as every second counts.

And so, the 35th President of the United States died as a result of blood loss so severe that a room full of doctors could do nothing to stop it, and of suffocation, for which the tracheotomy came too late. Strangely enough, the very first president of the United States, George Washington, died in a similar way, though in his case the loss of blood was caused by his doctors, who also allowed him to suffocate by refusing to perform a tracheotomy.

Washington's final hours are described in detail by an eyewitness, his personal secretary Colonel Tobias Lear. On Friday 13

December 1799, Washington had woken up with a sore throat. The day before, he had ridden through the snow on his horse. He was hoarse and coughing a lot. And yet, he still went out on his plantation in the cold winter weather. That night, he awoke with a high fever. He could hardly talk and began to have difficulty breathing. He was unable to swallow and became increasingly agitated. He tried to gargle with vinegar, but almost choked on it. On the Saturday morning, despite his wife's vigorous protests, he ordered his overseer to bleed him. But he felt no better and three doctors were called, James Craik, Gustavus Richard Brown and Elisha Cullen Dick. They bled the president several times, taking almost two and a half litres of blood in less than sixteen hours! Washington was eventually so weak that he could no longer sit upright, a position that is very important to breathe properly. Towards the evening, his breathing became increasingly laborious. He must have had a throat infection, causing his epiglottis to swell so much that it threatened to close off his windpipe. That makes the patient feel that he may suffocate at any moment, usually an extremely alarming experience. But Washington, who had by now lost nearly half of his blood, remained relatively calm. Dr Dick, the youngest of the three, wanted to perform a tracheotomy to save him but the other two, Craik and Brown, thought it too risky and refused to allow it. Washington died at ten o'clock in the evening, exhausted by the severe loss of blood and asphyxiated by a throat infection. He was sixty-eight years old.

It is no longer always necessary to perform a tracheotomy to alleviate an acute breathing problem. It was replaced by intubation – the insertion of a breathing tube into the windpipe via the mouth – around the beginning of the twentieth century. The breathing tube is one of the most successful life-saving devices in modern medicine. It is a simple, disposable plastic tube, flexible, about 1 centimetre in diameter and 30 centimetres long. There is a small balloon around the end, which is blown up once the tube has passed between the vocal cords and into the windpipe. That creates an airtight seal between the lungs and the respiratory machine to which the tube can be connected. This method is not only used to alleviate breathing problems, but also for respiration during general anaesthesia for operations. Effective intubation with a breathing tube in the patient's windpipe has become a basic condition of every large-scale operation. In the rare cases that intubation is not successful and the patient threatens to suffocate, a tracheotomy can always be used as a last resort.

The events of Friday 22 November 1963 would pursue Malcolm Perry for the rest of his life. He had been a surgeon for just two months when the dramatic events unfolded and he had a very busy few days. But it was far from over: Perry was called immediately to the operating theatre to operate on Governor Connally, and two days later he was there again, with his hands in Lee Harvey Oswald's abdomen, trying to stop arterial haemorrhaging.

3

Wound Healing

The Royal Prepuce: Abraham and King Louis XVI

A N OLD MAN hears a voice. He picks up a stone and strikes his penis to remove the prepuce, the foreskin. Then he does the same to his son and slaves. The men must have found the operation too painful as, shortly afterwards, it is decreed that circumcision is best not performed on adults but on male babies, on the eighth day after their birth.

The old man was Abraham. This story is told in chapter 17 of the Book of Genesis. Why he would do something so remarkable to himself can be explained not only historically, sociologically, anthropologically and theologically, but also surgically. At that moment, the old man had not successfully fathered a child for the past thirteen years. Throughout this whole chapter from Genesis it is clear that Abraham and his wife, Sarah, now both quite elderly, would still like to have a child of their own, but are having no luck. Could Abraham's foreskin have something to do with that?

There is an illness that can make sexual intercourse quite painful for a male: phimosis, a constriction of the foreskin caused by a chronic infection between the foreskin and the glans. The people of Abraham lived in the desert somewhere between Ur and the Mediterranean Sea. It was very dry and dust clouded up with every step they made. The robes they wore in those days were open from below and they wore nothing underneath them, so

the dust could go everywhere. Moreover, they had little understanding of hygiene. Genesis repeatedly speaks of people washing
themselves with water, but that is limited to the feet. Water was
scarce in the desert and needed for cattle. So there was probably
not enough to wash yourself daily. It is therefore not surprising
that the tradition of circumcision mainly prevailed – and still
does – among people who lived in the desert, not only in central
Asia – as with Abraham, the Jews and the Muslims – but also
among the Aboriginals in Australia and various African peoples.

Phimosis primarily becomes a problem during an erection, as
the glans is obstructed and the foreskin may tear. The movements
associated with sexual intercourse exacerbate the symptoms,
making it increasingly difficult to bring the act to a satisfactory
conclusion. Can this make a man so desperate, especially if he
passionately wants to found a long lineage, that he is willing to
remove the most logical cause of the problem – his foreskin – by
striking it with a stone? Don't most surgical operations have
similar origins? If you are sick to death of a pustule or an abscess
and the pain is keeping you from sleeping, you cut it open. If
the persistent throbbing, thumping pain of an infected tooth is
becoming unbearable, you rip it out. If a bladder stone is driving
you to distraction, you cut it out. If your foreskin is spoiling your
attempts at procreation, you strike it off with a stone. In any case,
shortly after this surgical operation, Abraham's wish is fulfilled.
In Genesis 21, Sarah gives birth to a son, Isaac.

What generally happens after circumcision is the theme of a
Bible story that reaches its climax in Genesis 34, verses 24 and
25. We are now three generations further. The sons of Jacob
promise not to avenge the defiling of their sister Dinah by a man
called Shichem, a Hivite, if all male Hivites allow themselves to
be circumcised. The Hivites, who were probably in the minority,
are more than happy that this will put an end to the matter and
agree. But they make the terrible mistake of all being circumcised

at the same time. That is not smart, as Jacob's sons are clearly better informed of the normal post-operative course than the Hivites. The same things happen after every operation – including a circumcision – with the same symptoms occurring.

During a surgical operation, the nerve fibres in the skin are stimulated directly. That means that the operation is immediately very painful. Not much later, after the knife – or stone – has been put aside, the initial pain ebbs away almost completely. The body has now started the healing process. In the first phase, the damage caused to the tissues is repaired by means of an inflammation. This is performed by special cells, called macrophages ('big eaters'), which clear away all the debris. As a result of this inflammation, some three hours after the operation, the tissue begins to swell, causing pain again, but this time less severe. The wound is a little swollen, a little red and a little warm. In hygienic conditions, that's as far as it goes. The inflammation disappears after a few days, and the pain with it. Cells known as fibroblasts ('fibre-makers') are now carried to the area of the wound and start to make connective tissue, ultimately forming the scar. This is called healing by primary intention (*per primam* in Latin) and usually lasts eight to fourteen days, depending on the depth of the wound.

However, in less hygienic circumstances, such as those described in the book of Genesis, bacteria in the wound will benefit from the damaged tissues, multiplying and attracting a second wave of inflammation cells. White blood cells, or leucocytes, try to destroy the bacteria. This leads to the formation of pus – a soup of harmful bacteria, dead leucocytes and damaged tissue. The wound becomes crimson, swollen and hot. In such circumstances, after an initial phase in which the pain is mild and bearable, there will be a new wave of excruciating pain, typically on the second day after the operation. Because, in biblical times, the day of an event was also counted, the second day after an operation was described

Inflammation

Inflammation is our body's reaction to something that should not be there. It is a varied and complex reaction performed by various kinds of cells, releasing a large number of substances, all of which either cause another reaction or serve as a signal for other cells. Through this complex process, an inflammation reaction can take various forms, depending on its cause. A sprained ankle, toothache, eczema, diarrhoea, AIDS, a smoker's cough, warts, an infected wound, the rejection of a transplanted kidney, hay fever, a malfunctioning thyroid gland, dandruff, typhoid, asthma, clogged-up arteries and mosquito bites are all forms of inflammation where a different aspect of the reaction comes to the fore. The local symptoms of inflammation can be summarised in five indications: *rubor* (redness), *calor* (heat), *dolor* (pain), *tumor* (swelling) and *functio laesa* (loss of function). Two kinds of cells are essential to an inflammation: macrophages (large cells called in to clear away the debris resulting from damaged cells) and lymphocytes (small cells that can recognise components of a foreign substance and manufacture antibodies to fight them). An allergy is an inflammatory reaction to a foreign substance that gets out of hand. An attack by intruders (a virus, bacteria or parasite) invokes an inflammation that we call an infection. If inflammation cells mistakenly see parts of our own bodies as foreign, the result is an autoimmune disease. An example is rheumatism, where parts of the joints are attacked by inflammation.

as the third day (just as Christ is described as having risen on the third day, while Easter Sunday is actually the second day after Good Friday).

That is why all the Hivites were in bed in terrible pain on the third day after their circumcision. With sharp surgical insight, Simeon and Levi – two of Jacob's sons – had counted on that.

They sneaked into the city with their swords drawn and slaughtered their defenceless patients in cold blood.

What happens to the operation wounds of patients who survive beyond the third day? As long as the wound is open and not too dirty and the tissue is not too badly damaged, the body is capable of fighting the infection. The pus can drip out of the wound and the bacteria are driven away from the healthy tissue, allowing the wound to heal. Until the mid-nineteenth century, surgical wounds were therefore always left open, because wound infections were inevitable. This is known as healing by secondary intention (*per secundam*). The wound gradually fills with granulating tissue and the skin grows over the wound from the edges until it is completely closed. Secondary healing can take a few weeks to several months, depending on the size of the wound.

In any case, we can conclude from both of these Bible stories that circumcision – at least at an adult age and in less than clean circumstances – is not a painless experience. It is not surprising that, several centuries later, the head of public relations of a young new religion pulled out all the stops to have circumcision removed as one of the requirements for men wishing to join the club. If St Paul had not put this point high on the agenda, Christendom would never have progressed much further than a Jewish splinter group. No adult Roman or Greek would have considered having himself circumcised. In the second century AD, the Roman emperor Hadrian (the one who had a wall named after him in Britain) issued a decree banning the practice. This led to two reactions, both politically and surgically: one progressive, the other reactionary.

Until then, circumcision had entailed cutting off only that part of the foreskin that could be pulled past the glans. This was known as the *mashuk* method. Partly in response to Hadrian's decree, Simon bar Kochba led the third Jewish rebellion against the Roman occupiers and propagated, by way of provocation, the *periah* method, fully exposing the glans. That entailed removing the rest of the foreskin by cutting around the base of the glans (this is the origin of the word circumcise, meaning 'to cut around'). Many of Bar Kochba's supporters had themselves re-circumcised during the revolt and full circumcision became the standard method.

Just as re-circumcision was a political statement, the reverse operation was also available to those with less fervent political views. Anyone who had been circumcised but did not want to join the Jewish revolt could have their foreskin repaired and remain an obedient citizen of the Roman Empire. The operation, known as epispasm, was apparently performed with some regularity, since the Roman encyclopaedist Celsus described it as early as the first century in his book *De Medicina*. It was an ingenious and, according to Celsus, not even very painful method of reconstructing the foreskin.

All you needed to perform it was a knife and a toothpick. An incision was made around the base of the penis. The skin was then slid forwards over the shaft like a sheath, so that the end could be pulled over the glans to form, as it were, a new foreskin. The skin would be held in place by the wooden stick until the gaping circular wound around the base was completed healed. It was an ingenious operation because the patient's urine did not come into contact with the open wound: an excellent example of the optimal use of secondary healing in times of limited hygiene.

Several centuries later, a new religion emerged in the same region. Although, these days, circumcision seems irrevocably linked to Islam, there is no mention of it in the Koran and it is not considered an obligation for Muslims. It is more a tradition. The thinking is that a father wishes his sons to look the same as he does.

In the dark ages that followed, Western civilisation lost its way.

While philosophers in antiquity spent their time thinking about noble questions like the essence of being, the ideal form of state and ethics, the great medieval thinkers concerned themselves with the issue of the foreskin. If Jesus genuinely ascended to heaven in physical form on Ascension Day, what happened to the foreskin that had been cut off when he was child? Did it, as the Greek scholar Leo Allatius claimed, make the journey to heaven independently?

Although the Vatican took no official standpoint on this issue, tour operators *avant la lettre* were keen to take advantage of the possibility that the holy foreskin was still somewhere on earth. Claiming to possess a sacred relic was an assured source of income for a town or village. Pilgrims were Europe's first tourists and tourism was a lucrative business, even back then. Cologne had the three kings, Constantinople the hand of John the Baptist, Trier the holy robe and Bruges the holy blood, while the sacred cross was splintered across the whole continent. After the small town of Charroux in France claimed to possess the foreskin of Christ, this mother of all relics turned up in a dozen other places in Europe. Even Antwerp had it. The last remaining foreskin was stolen from the small Italian village of Calcata in 1983.

Legend has it that the French royal family is directly descended via Charlemagne from Jesus of Nazareth, and therefore from Abraham as well. Christ's last royal descendant was therefore Louis XVI. It can be argued that Louis's foreskin played a decisive role in the advent of the French Revolution, which – as is well known – was to cost him his life. Louis also probably suffered from phimosis.

On 16 May 1770, the young Louis Auguste, the dauphin of France, was married to the Austrian archduchess Marie-Antoinette. They were both still children; he was fifteen years old and she was fourteen. On his wedding night, he fell asleep and early the next morning went hunting. His grandfather King Louis XV, the nobles at the royal court, and all the citizens of France were concerned that young Louis's love life seemed unable to get off the ground. Marie-Antoinette was beautiful and willing, but had married the only Louis in the French dynasty who was not lusty and hot-blooded. Her Louis was apparently a listless and impotent boy who seemed unable to move beyond puberty. There was a rumour that the prince had a disorder of the genitals that prevented him from engaging in sexual intercourse and it was openly speculated that a simple operation might be required to remove the obstacle. Two months after Louis's marriage, he was examined by Dr Germain Pichault de La Martinière, who found no abnormalities that might warrant an operation.

When young Louis had still not fulfilled his marital obligations after two years, his grandfather summoned him so that he could inspect the prince's private parts in person. Louis explained that the sexual act caused him pain, making him afraid to continue. The king observed what he had already suspected, an abnormality of the penis, but did not go into any further detail. He referred his grandson to Dr Joseph-Marie-François de Lassone. Lassone examined the dauphin in 1773 and made an official statement that, on the contrary, Louis's sexual organs were well formed. He concluded that the prince's impotence was more likely caused by the ignorance and awkwardness of the young couple. It was, however, widely believed that Louis had an overly tight foreskin that restricted his natural desires.

In 1774, the old king died and the impotent prince became King Louis XVI. That made the problem more urgent. The non-existent sex life of the young royal couple became a public matter discussed and gossiped about at court and in the city. France was buzzing with rhymes, jokes and songs about the king's assumed phimosis. On 15 January 1776, Louis XVI finally consulted a surgeon, Jacques-Louis Moreau, in the Hôtel-Dieu in Paris.

Marie-Antoinette later wrote to her mother that the surgeon had given the same advice as all the other doctors: that the problem would right itself without an operation. Louis just had to keep trying.

Moreau was right, as his colleague Lassone had been. We now know that phimosis at a young age is often cured by spontaneous nocturnal erections and sexual activity, and that an operation is only necessary in the most serious cases. Unfortunately, there are no further details of the findings of this eighteenth-century surgeon, but the fact that the king went to a hospital to consult a surgeon rather than just calling a doctor to visit him at home, suggests that there was something seriously wrong with him; that his foreskin probably was at least a little constricted. But it seems that Louis did nothing.

In 1777, Marie-Antoinette's brother came to visit with his entourage to try to sort out the matter. He apparently gave his brother-in-law a good talking to and put Lassone back on the job. This time there was no official report, but it did produce results. A few weeks later, in August of the same year, Louis and Marie-Antoinette were delighted. This time, it seemed to have worked. Dr Lassone was asked to confirm it officially: after seven years, the marriage had been consummated and the encounter in the royal bed had lasted an hour and a quarter. Marie-Antoinette wrote to her mother about the intense pleasure it had given her. The following year, she was pregnant and on 19 December 1778, she gave birth to their daughter, Marie-Thérèse.

It is tempting to compare this story with what happened to Abraham, but there is no official evidence of Louis undergoing a circumcision or any other operation on his foreskin. Yet it may be no coincidence that Dr Lassone was something of an expert in the surgical treatment of phimosis. He had even developed his own method for performing the operation, which he did not describe until much later, in 1786. It involved the smallest possible intervention, making only a few shallow scratches across the foreskin, rather than cutting it open completely, so that it could be pulled more easily over the glans. In this way, the foreskin was preserved completely intact without being deformed. Is it possible that Lassone performed this minor operation on Louis?

Because no clear – surgical – explanation was given for Marie-Antoinette's sudden pregnancy, the people of France most likely believed that she had committed adultery. Later, too, the royal couple rarely shared their marital bed and Marie-Antoinette was seen with other men. Before long, the French Revolution broke out and Louis and his wife were taken prisoner. What finally happened to them in 1793 is history. They had four children in total, of whom only the eldest, Marie-Thérèse, survived the Revolution.

According to an estimate by the World Health Organisation, in the year 2006 some 665 million men and boys underwent circumcision. Although a single foreskin weighs only a few grams, this means that hundreds of tons of foreskin are cut away every year. An estimated 30 per cent of the world's current population has been circumcised. That makes circumcision without doubt the most widely performed operation, not only now, but of all time.

In historic times, the foreskin was perhaps rightly considered unhygienic. In Arabic, the word for circumcision literally means 'cleaning'. In modern times, however, the removal of the foreskin no longer has any demonstrable medical benefits. And, although today's surgical conditions mean that complications are now rare, serious bleeding and infections do still occur, sometimes with fatal consequences. From a surgical perspective, it is unacceptable to conduct a futile operation on children who are too young to ask if they approve of their foreskin being removed for ever.

For men and boys suffering from a genuine phimosis, as was perhaps the case with Abraham and Louis XVI, full circumcision is not actually necessary. In the case of children, the problem often rights itself or is cured with a salve. If not, it can be put right with a much less invasive operation than circumcision. For adults, too, there are various methods that leave the function of the foreskin intact, as with the operation devised by Lassone.

4

Shock

The Lady and the Anarchist: Empress Sisi

I N MEDICAL TERMS, shock means a failure of the blood's circulatory system. A constant flow of blood is essential for every organ in our bodies. And that requires sufficient blood pressure. Shock is what happens if our blood pressure falls so low that our organs do not receive sufficient oxygen, and it has catastrophic consequences.

Not all organs can last equally long without a sufficient supply of blood. The brain and the kidneys will be the first to fail. Then our consciousness decreases and our urine production stops. That is followed by the intestines, lungs, liver and heart. A state of shock that persists for too long therefore leads to multiple organ failure (MOF). To understand the mechanisms of shock, it is first important to know that the walls of the arteries in our bodies contain small muscles that allow the blood vessels to dilate or contract, known medically as vasodilation (widening of the blood vessel) and vasoconstriction (narrowing of the vessel). This is one way in which our bodies can regulate blood pressure. The heart can also affect blood pressure by beating slower or faster or by pumping more strongly.

The circulatory system comprises three essential components: the heart, the blood and the blood vessels. The heart pumps the blood through the vessels. Failure of the circulatory system can be caused by any of these three components, resulting in different kinds of shock. Firstly, there is cardiogenic shock (literally 'caused by the heart'), which may occur because of a heart attack, a faulty heart valve or an injury to the heart. Secondly, there is hypovolemic shock (literally 'with too little volume'), which is caused by insufficient blood being pumped around the system, for example as a result of dehydration or bleeding. In both cases, the blood vessels will constrict (vasoconstriction) to keep the blood pressure up. This reflex is triggered by nerves that run to the blood vessels, and by adrenaline released by the adrenal glands. By contrast, the third form of shock (septic shock) occurs when the blood vessels dilate excessively as a result of toxic substances paralysing and damaging the vessel wall. That causes the blood pressure to fall, the mechanism that regulates the blood pressure to stop working and fluid to leak to the surrounding tissues. The toxic substances that invoke septic shock come mostly from bacteria or dead tissue resulting, for example, from burns, gangrene or blood poisoning.

An operation can cause all three kinds of shock: cardiogenic by overtaxing the heart, hypovolemic through blood loss, or septic shock as a result of damaged tissue and infection. Shock can sometimes be treated surgically by, for example, stopping massive haemorrhaging, draining pus from an infection, or cutting away dead or damaged tissue. In this chapter we look at the story of an exceptional woman with a case of shock, unfortunately with an unhappy ending.

On 10 September 1898 an Italian anarchist named Luigi Lucheni attacked the Austrian empress, Elisabeth, commonly known as Sisi, by thrusting a small, triangular file into her chest. But when the sixty-year-old simply got to her feet again, straightened her hat and calmly continued on her way, he must have watched the aftermath of his assault with astonishment. It was only later, when two police officers arrested him for murder, that he realised he had apparently succeeded, after all.

Lucheni would testify that his main motive was to kill someone royal, no matter who. His victim had been spotted by paparazzi some days previously in the Hôtel Beau Rivage on the shores of Lake Geneva, and Lucheni had read about it in the newspapers. The empress was in many ways the Lady Diana of her time. Not only because both their deaths were indirectly caused by paparazzi but, like Diana, she was a princess who married the handsome prince of an important country, just as in a fairy tale. In 1854, when she married the twenty-three-year-old Emperor Franz Joseph at the age of sixteen, she became both Empress and Queen of the mighty Habsburg Empire, which extended from Russia to Milan and from Poland to Turkey. The popularity of the beautiful Empress Elisabeth of Austria soared again in the 1950s, with the release of the 'Sisi' films, in which she was played by the beautiful Romy Schneider. The real Sisi's life, however, was much less like a fairy tale than the film suggests. Elisabeth suffered from an eating disorder, which we would now call anorexia nervosa. In her youth, she weighed only 46 kilograms. In addition, she always wore a tight corset to preserve her wasp waist, which was less than 50 centimetres in circumference – the equivalent of a diameter of only 16 centimetres! She was wearing one of these contraptions when she left her hotel in Geneva on that day to take the steamboat to Montreux.

Her lady-in-waiting Countess Irma Sztáray de Sztára et Nagymihály, who accompanied her, stated later that, as they were walking along the waterfront, her Royal Highness was suddenly knocked to the ground by a man. But she stood up again quickly, said that she was fine, and carried on walking so as not to miss the boat. Once on board, she became pale and fainted, but regained consciousness rapidly and asked what had happened. The boat was by then in open water and the captain was asked to turn about. To relieve her mistress's distress, the lady-in-waiting loosened Elisabeth's tight corset, at which the empress passed out again. Only then did the countess see a small spot of blood the size of a silver coin on the dying empress's undergarment. The boat moored and members of the crew carried Elisabeth, who was probably already dead, back to the hotel on an improvised stretcher made of two oars. In the hotel, the death of the empress was confirmed by a doctor cutting open an artery in her arm. No blood came out. It was ten past two in the afternoon.

An autopsy revealed a stab wound 8.5 centimetres deep near the fourth rib on the left side, which extended through the lung and across the whole width of the heart, causing internal bleeding. How could someone with such severe wounds through their heart still have got to the Montreux boat?

Our bodies possess a number of regulatory and reserve systems to provide a first response to serious problems. The fact that the sixty-year-old Elisabeth was able to survive for that long with a punctured heart is, first and foremost, a sign that she was generally in good health. Sisi was a healthy woman. She was not overweight, had grown up in the mountains, had never smoked and had ridden horses her whole life. That healthy condition explains why all the organs and systems in her body were functioning well when the attack took place.

Elisabeth was of course alarmed immediately after the incident. And she was afraid of missing the boat. This state of agitation stimulated a part of her nervous system known as the sympathetic nervous system, which had immediately made her body alert. Her heartbeat increased, her muscles received more blood and her adrenal glands were activated to release adrenaline into the bloodstream. The name 'adrenal' comes from the location of these two small glands, on top of (Latin 'ad') each kidney (Latin 'ren'). High concentrations of adrenaline therefore flowed through her blood, strengthening the effects of the sympathetic nervous system. This must have given her enough energy to get to the boat on time.

Sisi did not faint until she was on board. The cause was shock, a sudden fall in blood pressure. The first organ to suffer from low blood pressure is the one that needs the most oxygen, the brain. That is why a reduction in consciousness – fainting – is often the first sign of shock. The fall in blood pressure may have already been caused by the loss of blood from the heart – in other words, bleeding leading to hypovolemic shock – but that is not very likely. The internal blood loss from a punctured heart would, after all, have been so severe that Elisabeth would never have been able to walk another hundred metres. The loss of blood therefore had to be restricted by something and the shock must have been caused by something else.

Sisi had developed a cardiac tamponade. The word tamponade comes from the French *tamponner*, meaning 'to tamp' or 'plug up'. With a cardiac tamponade, blood from a wound to the heart accumulates in the pericardium, the rigid sac that surrounds (*peri*) the heart. As Luigi's file was quite thin, the hole in the pericardium was too small for blood to escape easily. Therefore, the loss of blood was initially limited, but as it accumulated in the pericardium, the heart had less and less room and came under increasing pressure. In this way, an apparently small loss of blood could have serious consequences for the functioning of the heart.

The shock was thus initially caused by the constriction of the heart and not by the loss of blood. A constricted heart cannot beat properly, so that Sisi first experienced cardiogenic shock. As a result of the reduced functioning of the heart, the blood pressure falls. That low blood pressure is registered at various points in the body. There are sensors on both sides of the arteries in the neck, which record low blood pressure and pass the information on to the brain stem. There the sympathetic nervous system is activated, contracting the blood vessels throughout the body to boost the blood pressure. The kidneys also register low blood pressure and temporarily retain the body's reserves of fluid. If you could have asked her, Elisabeth would have said that she was terribly thirsty.

Specialisation

If you tell people you are a surgeon, they usually ask 'What kind of surgeon?' Many do not seem to know that being a surgeon is a profession in itself, and that you can therefore be a general surgeon. Medical specialisations can be divided into medicine (the 'non-cutting' professions) – which includes internal medicine, paediatrics, neurology, psychiatry and pathology – and surgery (the 'cutting' professions). For many centuries, surgeons applied themselves to all aspects of surgery, but in the twentieth century a number of specialisations went their own way. Gynaecologists operate on the female reproductive organs, and urologists on the kidneys, the urinary tract and the male reproductive organs. Cosmetic surgery, reconstructive surgery, microsurgery and hand surgery are all performed by plastic surgeons. Neurosurgeons operate on the brain, the spine and the nerves. Orthopaedic surgeons focus on the musculo-skeletal system, while ear, nose and throat specialists need no further explanation. The rest can be classified horizontally, by theme, or vertically, by organ system. Horizontally, there is traumatology (operations following accidents), oncological surgery (cancer operations) and paediatric surgery (operations on children). Vertically, there is cardiac surgery (on the heart), thoracic surgery (the lungs), vascular surgery (the blood vessels) and gastrointestinal or abdominal surgery (the organs in the abdomen). General surgery still embraces five of these components: traumatology, oncological surgery, thoracic surgery, gastrointestinal or abdominal surgery, and vascular surgery. Paediatric surgery and cardiac surgery are separate specialisations. In some countries, breast cancer is not treated by a surgeon but a gynaecologist and traumatology by orthopaedic surgeons. There are also a number of 'super-specialisations' within general surgery, including head and neck surgery, transplant surgery and bariatric surgery.

The lady-in-waiting reported that Sisi had become remarkably pale. The normal pink colour of the skin is caused by the flow of blood. If that pink becomes paler, it can be due to anaemia resulting from a severe loss of blood. But the contraction of the blood vessels also reduces the flow of blood in the skin, so the paleness that afflicted the empress when she fainted was consistent with cardiogenic shock. Contraction of the blood vessels can also make you go pale from fright. The lady-in-waiting probably looked as pale her mistress.

A cardiac tamponade reduces the functioning of the heart in two ways. The heart is a hollow muscle that dilates to fill itself with blood and then contracts to pump it out again. In the event of a cardiac tamponade, the heart muscle can pump the blood out, but is unable to refill itself sufficiently because of the pressure in the pericardium. Consequently, with the next heartbeat, there is less blood to pump away. But something else happens, too. The strength of the heart muscle depends heavily on the heart being optimally filled. With a cardiac tamponade, the heart will therefore not only pump less amounts of blood but also with less power.

Elisabeth fainted on the boat. Yet, shortly afterwards, she came round again in the arms of her lady-in-waiting. That is because, after fainting, she ended up lying horizontally. That increased the flow of blood from the legs and the abdomen to the heart, as it no longer had to fight gravity and flow upwards. As a result, Sisi's heart was able to fill up with more blood, and thus pump more blood around and, above all, more strongly. Several minutes passed. It can be assumed that, during that time, a large volume of blood did actually flow through the small hole in the pericardium into the chest cavity. This was later confirmed by the autopsy. So how was it possible that Sisi was still alive and was able to talk to her lady-in-waiting?

The answer to this medical puzzle is probably her corset. Because her abdomen and pelvis were compressed by the tight corset, there was relatively more blood in her upper body than normal. When the lady-in-waiting released the corset, this reserve of blood was once again able to flow throughout Elisabeth's whole body, leaving relatively less blood close to her heart.

After the corset was opened, therefore, the heart no longer filled with enough blood. The body had no more emergency plans left to call upon. The blood vessels were already contracted as far as possible and the heartbeat had reached its maximum rate, at Elisabeth's age probably around 160 beats a minute. She may also have been struck by one last catastrophe. As a result of the shock, her heart itself could have received insufficient oxygen. The electrical circuit of the heart muscle is the first to notice this problem. Normally, the circuit ensures that the heartbeat is regular and coordinated, so that the heart can function optimally. But a lack of oxygen can cause a fatal fault in this circuit. Elisabeth's heart would have started to fibrillate, contracting chaotically with no effect at all, causing her death.

If Elisabeth had made it to a hospital instead of the boat, it is doubtful whether they would have taken the chance of operating on her. Professor Theodor Billroth, the world-renowned surgeon who had called the shots in Vienna for many years, had died four years previously, but his words were still seen as the gold standard in surgery. He had been very resolute about heart surgery. Without a single ounce of evidence to support his statement, this bully of a professor had left the surgical world cowering under the threat: 'Surgeons who attempt to operate on the heart can no longer count on the respect of their colleagues.' Only two years after Billroth's death did a surgeon, Ludwig Rehn, dare to stitch a stab wound in the heart for the first time. Although his patient, whose heart had been pierced by a sword, survived the operation, it would be many years before surgeons would begin to explore the field of cardiac surgery.

Today, thanks to that breathtaking new branch of surgery,

Elisabeth would have a greater chance of surviving a stab wound to the heart. It is only 2.5 kilometres from where she was attacked, the Quai du Mont-Blanc, to what is now Geneva University Hospital. An ambulance could be on the spot within ten minutes. A happy ending would, however, require bystanders on the quay or the jetty to start treating her shock immediately. The lady-in-waiting would have to start CPR as soon as Sisi fainted after her corset was opened. The rhythmic up and down movement of the sternum turns the whole chest into one large pump. This would have kept Elisabeth's blood pressure up at a safe level. Performing CPR is very tiring and the lady-in-waiting's pale face would soon become scarlet. Other people would have to take over and keep going until the ambulance arrived. The ambulance crew would then immediately insert a breathing tube into the windpipe and a needle into a vein to introduce litres of fluid directly into the blood vessels – the most effective way to treat shock. If the heart was fibrillating, they could use a defibrillator to deliver an electric shock to normalise the heart-beat. They would also administer adrenaline through the intravenous needle and oxygen through the breathing tube, and the empress would be made ready for transport to hospital. In the meantime, at the hospital, an operating team would be called together and, in the operating theatre, the heart–lung machine would be prepared. Once she was on the operating table, her sternum would be sawn open vertically to connect the input and output tubes of the heart–lung machine in the open chest cavity. The machine would take over the pumping action of her heart and the respiratory function of her lungs. The surgeons would pour ice water into her chest cavity to stop her heart and cool it off, and the operation could start. But, in 1898, that was all far into the future.

Sisi was the victim of the 'propaganda of the deed', a bizarre philosophy associated with anarchism. In that respect, she was in good company: between 1881 and 1913, a series of public figures – including the Russian Tsar Alexander II, the Italian King Umberto I, the French President Sadi Carnot, the Greek King George I and the American President William McKinley were assassinated by anarchists. Luigi Lucheni was given a life sentence and committed suicide in his cell in 1910. His head was saved, in the interests of science. It was not until 2000 that it was decided that this rogue's head was of little scientific interest and it was buried in the Vienna Central Cemetery, where Beethoven and Billroth also enjoy eternal rest. As was customary among deceased imperial and royal Habsburgs, Sisi's body was interred in the Capuchin Crypt in Vienna. Unlike the deceased members of her in-laws' family, however, her intestines were not interred separately in the crypt beneath St Stephen's Cathedral and her pierced heart was not placed in a silver goblet in the Augustinian Church. Luigi's file can be seen in the Sisi Museum in the Hofburg palace complex. The dress – with the hole made by the file – is on display at the national museum in Budapest. But without the corset.

5

Obesity

Popes: From Peter to Francis

A REMARKABLE MEDICAL CONCLUSION can be drawn from the long list of 305 popes and antipopes that have graced Roman Catholic history to the present day. Their five year survival rate after being ordained was only 54 per cent. One in five did not even survive their first year. Being elected as pope therefore has a rather sombre prognosis, though some were so old when they took high office that it is no surprise they did not keep it for long. Clement XII was the oldest, elected in 1730 at the age of seventy-nine, yet he was pope for ten years. In 1975, Pope Paul VI set the maximum age at which a cardinal could still be elected pope at eighty years old. Benedict XVI was only two years short of this upper limit when he was elected in 2005.

A common cause of death among popes in the past was malaria, which was prevalent in the marshes around Rome. It mainly affected those from outside Italy, who were not accustomed to the local climate and the mosquitoes that thrived in it.

The death of a pope was often kept under wraps – and not only in the distant past. The details of the death of sixty-five-year-old Pope John Paul I in 1978, only thirty-three days after he was elected, are still shrouded in mystery. Still relatively young for a pope, he was found dead in his bed one morning. A post-mortem was never carried out and the accusations of foul play flew back and forth in the Italian and Vatican banking world. Only nine popes have held the pontificate for a shorter time.

Sisinnius died after twenty days in 708 and Theodore II lasted for three weeks in 897. Leo V managed a whole month in 903, Celestine IV only seventeen days in 1241, Pius III twenty-six days in 1503, Marcellus II twenty-two days in 1555, Urban VII twelve days in 1590 and Leo XI twenty-seven days in 1605. Boniface VI, pope in the turbulent ninth century, died after only fifteen days, allegedly after 'an attack of gout'. He may, however, have been poisoned by his successor Stephen VI, the malignant pope who dug up the corpse of Boniface's predecessor in 896 to bring it to trial. In 752, Stephen II did not even make it to his ordination, dying three days after being elected. The only Englishman to occupy the papal throne, Adrian IV, died within five years, choking on a fly in his wine in 1159. His namesake Adrian VI from Utrecht – the only Dutch pope in Roman Catholic history – survived twelve months in Rome, dying there in 1523.

From a surgical point of view, the medical histories of a number of popes are worth mentioning. In 1404, Boniface IX is alleged to have died of stones, possibly in his gall bladder, after being ill for two days. Alexander VIII succumbed in 1691 to the effects of gangrene in his leg. Pius VII, who had the misfortune to be pope during the time of Napoleon Bonaparte, died forty-five days after falling in his bedroom and fracturing his hip. At the end of the last century, in his apartment in the Vatican, Paul VI underwent a secret operation on his prostate via the urethra. The equipment purchased especially for the operation was later donated to a missionary hospital in a developing country. In 2009, Benedict XVI broke his wrist while on holiday, but that could be treated with a simple forearm plaster. He later had two small operations to implant a pacemaker to correct heart arrhythmia. And Jorge Bergoglio, the current pope Francis, had the upper lobe of his right lung removed at the age of twenty-one to treat bronchiectasis, dilations of the airways caused in the lung tissue following pneumonia.

There was also a pope who was a surgeon himself. Pope John
XXI was a professor of medicine in his home country of Portugal
before being elected to the pontificate in 1276. He must therefore
also have been active as a surgeon. During his term of office, he
continued his study of philosophy and medicine in Italy. He
wrote a book on the medical and surgical sciences, a standard
work in medieval times, with the dramatic title *Thesaurus Pauperum*,
the 'treasure chest for the poor'. It was a kind of almanac, intended
to make the achievements in healthcare available to the common
folk, so that they could also benefit from them (if they could
read, of course). Doctors had anxiously protected their knowledge
for many centuries, for fear that their patients would no longer
pay for their services. And perhaps also not to be caught out, as
that knowledge actually did not amount to much. The pope's
book was thus mainly an extensive collection of home remedies
and old wives' tales. It offered cures for all kinds of complaints,
surgical operations and recipes for preparing medicines. He even
described several forms of contraception and ways to abort a
foetus. Anyone who claims that contraception and abortion are
incompatible with the prevailing views of the Vatican should take
a look at this book by Pope John XXI.

But all that rummaging around in old books was considered
suspect. As a bona fide medieval professor, John must have famil-
iarised himself with alchemy and have messed around with
alembics and astrolabes which would have aroused suspicion,
especially in the thirteenth century, that the Pope was not what
he seemed. Rumours soon began that this strange (foreign!)
professor was actually a magician. Pope John XXI would be
irrevocably punished by God, as in the spring of 1277, the ceiling
of his workroom suddenly fell on his head. As he lay there, buried
beneath rubble and piles of heavy manuscripts, he allegedly just
about managed to utter 'My book! Who shall finish my book?'
Seriously hurt, he succumbed to his injuries six days later to

widespread agreement that this was a deserved punishment for messing around with black magic.

Operations and obesity

Bariatric surgery is the branch of gastrointestinal surgery concerned with obesity. The word 'bariatric' comes from the Greek *baros* (weight) and *iater* (doctor). It is a form of functional surgery and makes use of two kinds of operations. One reduces the size of the stomach, so that the patient eats less. This can be achieved by a gastric bypass, gastric banding or a sleeve gastrectomy. The second kind of operation, an intestinal bypass, reduces the functioning of the intestines so that less food is digested. There are also combinations of both methods. The gastric bypass, which has been conducted since 1969, is the most effective operation to reduce the size of the stomach. We now know that these operations can treat much more than obesity. They can also cure diabetes type 2, obstructive sleep apnoea syndrome (OSAS), high blood pressure and high cholesterol. Obesity is a known risk factor in all operations; the more overweight the patient, the more complications can occur. It is therefore to be expected that complications occur more often in bariatric surgery than with other forms of surgery. It has, however, become considerably safer since the introduction of laparoscopic (keyhole) surgery. Bariatric surgery is not a luxury − obesity is a serious threat to the patient's health and, to date, it is the only treatment for obesity that can give the patient high expectations of sustained weight loss.

A common weakness among popes throughout the centuries was gluttony. It is alleged, for example, that Pope Martin IV died in 1285 after gorging himself on Lake Bolsena eels fed with milk. Pope Innocent VIII was also immensely fat and slept the whole day. On top of that, he was certainly not a pleasant man. He was the pope who instigated the horrific witch-hunts that led to thousands of innocent women being burned alive. He eventually became so obese that he could no longer move and had to be breastfed by young women. You can imagine that the doctor who gave this advice had little trouble in retaining his post with the Holy See. For some incomprehensible reason, it was then decided to postpone the approaching end of this pope's worthless life by giving him a blood transfusion. Three healthy young Roman boys each gave their blood for a ducat, but it was to no avail. The pope and his three blood donors died and the story goes that the coins had to be wrenched from the balled fists of the young men.

Whether this was a blood transfusion as we now know it is not clear. Perhaps they simply gave the pope the blood to drink, let the boys bleed to death, and then the patient died anyway. But even if it was a vein-to-vein transfusion, the deaths of all four can be easily explained. After all, blood groups were not discovered until four hundred years later, in 1900, by Karl Landsteiner. There is little chance that Innocent had the rare blood group AB-positive, which would have protected him against an incorrect transfusion, while the chances that all three of the young men were O-negative, so that the pope could have successfully used their blood no matter what type he had, are even smaller.

Obesity, falling asleep during the day and an unpleasant humour are, in religious terms, a combination of three of the seven deadly sins – *gula* (gluttony), *acedia* (sloth) and *ira* (wrath) – but are compatible, in medical terms, with obstructive sleep apnoea syndrome (OSAS). OSAS is a sleeping sickness caused mostly by obesity whereby, at night, the breathing stops repeatedly for a short time (apnoea). This is usually accompanied by snoring. Because of this disruption of their nightly rest, sufferers are unable to sleep deeply enough to enter the necessary REM phase. That makes them sleepy, bad-tempered and remarkably lethargic during the day. They will also often feel hungry, exacerbating their obesity and therefore their sleeping problems. Charles Dickens described a character with exactly these symptoms in his 1837 novel *The Pickwick Papers*. Consequently, OSAS is also sometimes referred to as Pickwick syndrome.

Today OSAS can be treated effectively with a laparoscopic gastric bypass, a stomach-reducing operation that can break the vicious circle of lethargy, obesity and insomnia. It could have made a lot of difference in the case of Innocent VIII, as a fit, contented and effective world leader was exactly what the doctor ordered in those dark ages. If Innocent VIII did indeed suffer from OSAS, his death must be considered a genuine medical failure. Obstructive sleep apnoea syndrome can cause a chronic shortage of oxygen, stimulating the production of red blood cells. This results in an excessively high level of these cells in the blood rather than anaemia, meaning that you should definitely not give the patient a transfusion. Whatever the real cause may have been, Innocent's death in 1492 marked a fitting end to the dark Middle Ages.

In contrast to Innocent VIII, his grandson Giovanni di Lorenzo de' Medici, lord of Florence, represented the colourful highpoint in the history of the papacy. Giovanni, alias Pope Leo X, is reputed to have said when elected to the pontificate at the age of thirty-seven, 'since God has given us the papacy, let us enjoy it'. During his seven years in the office, he managed to work his way through 5 million ducats (the equivalent of hundreds of millions of euros!). He raised the money by selling indulgences to poor sinners and clerical positions to the highest bidders, and spent it on orgies, parties, art and an opulent lifestyle.

Like a number of other well-known figures from the Renaissance Leo X was homosexual. He suffered continually from fistula and fissures of the anus. That could be seen from the expression on his face when he rode through Rome on a snow-white horse with unprecedented pomp and circumstance on the day of his ordination as pope. His alleged lover was twenty-six-year-old Cardinal Alfonso Petrucci. Apparently, in 1516, the pope had had enough of Alfonso and came up with a scarcely credible story to rid himself of the young man. The pope was to undergo surgery on his anus by a surgeon called Vercelli. He claimed that Alfonso had bribed the surgeon to inject poison into his holiness's rear end during the operation – at least this is what the unfortunate Vercelli had confessed during his interrogation in the torture chamber. The surgeon was quartered, but that was only a triviality. Cardinal Alfonso was found guilty and condemned to death. The pope had his former boyfriend strangled with a red silk cord.

It was not so surprising that the Florentine pope had such a low regard for surgeons. Florence was a proverbial hotbed of sodomy. For many years, surgeons were obliged to report the anal complaints of their male patients to the city magistrates so that they – the patients – could be prosecuted.

Julius III was one of the most shamelessly gluttonous popes of all. Ironically, in the last few months of his life, he suffered from increasing problems with swallowing. Eventually he could not eat at all and, in 1555, he starved to death. These symptoms closely resemble those of cancer of the stomach or oesophagus. Malignant tumours where the oesophagus enters the stomach display typical symptoms and the prognosis is grim. The main problem is dysphagia, a medical term for difficulty with swallowing. While the growth is still small, it will cause problems with swallowing solid food, especially food like meat that is difficult to chew. The patient develops *horror carnis*, Latin for 'fear of meat'. Food gets stuck in the oesophagus, giving the sufferer bad breath, *foetor ex ore* (Latin for 'a smell from the mouth'). Swallowing becomes increasingly difficult and, within a few months, it is only possible to ingest liquid food. The rapidly growing cancerous tumour requires increasing energy and uses up the body's reserves of protein and fat. Exactly when the patient needs more nutrition, he is no longer able to eat. He becomes emaciated, and develops cachexia – severe malnutrition – which ultimately leads to death.

Four hundred years later, Angelo Roncalli became the kind-hearted and widely loved Pope John XXIII, who tried to steer the Catholic Church into the modern age in the 1960s by convening the Second Vatican Council. He, too, was seriously overweight. So much so in fact that they were unable to find anything to fit him when he was due to appear on the balcony of St Peter's after his election. He therefore had to wear a robe with the back cut open. The cheering crowd on the square noticed nothing out of the ordinary. This pontiff also succumbed to stomach cancer.

A tumour in the stomach does not usually cause problems with swallowing until a later stage, because the oesophagus is not affected. Yet *horror carnis*, the fear of meat, is typically one of the first symptoms of stomach cancer. In the stomach, the tumour is attacked by gastric juices. That causes an ulcer, which generates pain in the upper abdomen. The ulcer on the tumour can bleed, slowly, causing anaemia, or suddenly, leading to haematemesis (vomiting blood) and melena, a medical term for faeces that are coloured black due to blood in the intestines.

As the tumour becomes larger, the patient will – as with oesophageal cancer – find it increasingly difficult to eat. Undigested food will be vomited out, leading eventually to fatal cachexia. Pope John XXIII did not reach this stage. He was diagnosed with stomach cancer after undergoing a stomach X-ray to investigate the symptoms of anaemia. The diagnosis was kept secret as long as possible. More than two thousand bishops from around the world attended the Council. John was the centre of attention, while he must have continually suffered from pain and stomach problems. He experienced repeated stomach haemorrhaging and was hospitalised on several occasions. He died in 1963, at the age of eighty-one, from a perforated stomach. The ulcer in his tumour had eaten through the stomach wall.

If the stomach perforates, the contents of the stomach and gastric acid can enter the abdominal cavity and the patient feels a sudden, acute pain in the upper abdomen, like a stab wound. The peritonitis that always follows is a life-threatening condition that can only be treated with an emergency operation. The hole in the stomach must be closed or a piece of the stomach removed, and the abdominal cavity thoroughly rinsed with water. It was decided, however, not to perform this operation on the old pope. Medically and ethically, that was a wise decision. There was already no hope of recovery and this saved him from a miserable death from cachexia. Pope John XXIII survived another nine days with the peritonitis resulting from the stomach perforation. His body was laid to rest in an altar in St Peter's Basilica, embalmed in a glass coffin.

Pope John XXIII was canonised by one of his successors, Pope John Paul II. This popular Polish pope was, in surgical terms, the most interesting of all 305 pontiffs, in that he underwent the most operations.

6

Stoma

The Miracle Bullet: Karol Wojtyła

H<small>E WAS A</small> media superstar, completely different from his Italian predecessors: young, fond of sports, enthusiastic, smart and enterprising, and he would play a significant role in the fall of Communism in the Eastern bloc. On 13 May 1981 his popularity rose to unprecedented heights when he survived being shot in the abdomen. It was the second time he had been shot at. As a child, a friend had accidentally fired a gun, just missing him. This time, he was severely wounded. He was saved by Italian surgeons who, apparently, fought not only to save his life, but also over the operation itself.

Around five o'clock that afternoon, standing in the back of a white jeep, Pope John Paul II drove across St Peter's Square through a cheering crowd of some 20,000 people. The crowd included two Turks with guns and a bomb, Mehmet Ali Ağca and Oral Çelik. At 5.19 p.m., twenty-three-year-old Ağca fired his 9mm Browning pistol twice. He hit Ann Odre, a sixty-year-old American, in her chest, Rose Hill, a twenty-one-year-old woman from Jamaica in her left upper arm, and Karol Józef Wojtyła, the sixty-year-old pope, in his abdomen, from a distance of six metres. The Turk was overpowered by a nun called Sister Laetitia. Çelik did nothing. The popemobile raced out of the square through the screaming crowd. The severely injured pope was taken in an ambulance to the Gemelli Hospital, five kilometres away and the nearest university hospital in the city. On arrival, he was not taken to the emergency department, but to the papal suite on the tenth floor.

Duty surgeon Giovanni Salgarello found a small gunshot wound just to the left of the navel and other wounds on the right upper arm and left index finger. The patient was still alert for a short time and was given the last rites. When he lost consciousness and went into shock, the pope was moved to the operating department. He was placed under general anaesthesia at 6.04 p.m., three-quarters of an hour after being shot. While inserting a breathing tube via the mouth (intubation), the anaesthetist accidentally broke off one of the Holy Father's teeth. Salgarello disinfected the abdomen and covered the area around it with sterile drapes. He took a scalpel and was about to start the operation when his boss, Francesco Crucitti, stormed into the operating room. He had been in his private practice when he heard the news and had jumped into his car and sped through Rome, to arrive just in time to start the operation himself.

From the sparse information that the surgeons gave to the Italian media and with a little surgical imagination, it can be surmised that the operation proceeded as follows. Crucitti and Salgarello made a long incision along the centre line of the pope's abdomen from top to bottom. When the peritoneum, the membrane lining the abdominal cavity, was opened, blood streamed out. The pope's blood pressure had fallen far below the normal 100mm Hg to 70mm Hg. The surgeons scooped the largest clots of blood out with their hands, removed blood with a suction device, and applied pressure to the bleeding wounds with gauzes. It was later estimated that the pope had lost three litres of blood, but he was administered no less than ten units of A-negative blood during the operation, which suggests that he lost much more. The abdominal cavity contained not only blood but also stools. The surgeons felt along the whole length of the intestinal tract with their hands and discovered five holes in the small intestine and the mesentery, which attaches the small bowel to the back of the abdomen. They then placed clamps on all the bleeding wounds they could easily get at, but the abdominal cavity continued to fill with blood. It seemed to be coming from below. The operating table was tilted so the pope was lying with his head downwards. Using all four hands, the surgeons pushed the bowels as far upwards as possible, so that they could see the bottom of the abdominal cavity. That is where the major blood vessels to the legs are to be found. Because of the bleeding, it was not clear whether they were damaged, but somewhere deep down, Crucitti felt a hole as thick as his finger in the 'holy bone' or sacrum, the triangular bone at the base of the spine. He pressed it closed with his hand and the worst bleeding seemed to stop.

Crucitti filled the hole with sterile wax, so that he could inspect the area around it. The major blood vessels to and from the left leg were immediately next to the hole, but had not been damaged. That was a good sign and everyone around the operating table must have heaved a deep sigh of relief. The bleeding seemed under control.

It was a good moment to consult with the anaesthetic team at the head end of the table. They, too, had been busy. The lost blood was feverishly replenished with fluid and transfusions, and the pope's blood pressure and heart activity were closely monitored. There, too, everything seemed more or less under control. The patient was out of danger, for the time being.

So what happens next in such an operation? Usually, the surgeons would inspect the abdominal cavity again, make a plan, and set to work. First they would remove the clamps from the bleeding wounds one at a time and close them with absorbable sutures. The surgical assistant counts all the clamps, to make sure nothing gets left behind. Then the surgeons remove the gauzes one at a time from the abdominal cavity and check that the bleeding has stopped. In the meantime, a nurse counts and weighs the gauzes as they go in and out.

The surgeons examined the inside of the Holy Father's abdominal wall. The bullet hole was on the left. They checked the organs in the upper abdomen – the liver, the transverse part of the large intestine, the stomach and the spleen – and found them all intact. Then they looked at the kidneys: these, too, were undamaged. And then the whole length of the intestinal tract was inspected, metres of small intestine and metres of large intestine. There, in the lower left quadrant of the abdomen, they found a long tear in the sigmoid colon, the last part of the large intestine (named after the Greek letter sigma, because it is 'S' shaped). Now they could reconstruct the trauma exactly.

All of the holes they had found so far fitted a single, simple trajectory – from front left in the abdominal wall, through the small intestine and part of the large intestine, to the sacrum at the back. Had the bullet gone any further? Had anyone seen a bullet hole in the patient's back? 'Damn, has no one checked el Papa's back side?' must have resounded through the operating room. It was too late to turn him around now. They decided to take an X-ray at the end of the operation to see if a bullet was still lodged in the pope's sacrum or buttock.

They then removed the gauzes from the pelvis. It was reasonably dry. Though the hole in the sacrum was immediately next to the left iliac artery and vein (the large blood vessels to and from the left leg), they were undamaged. The left ureter, the tube that transports urine from the kidney to the bladder, was also intact. That was a stroke of luck. So now for the operation plan. The holes in the small intestine were no great problem. The surgeons decided to remove two pieces of small bowel and thus create two new connections. A small hole in the terminal ileum, the final part of the small intestine, was easily repaired. The tear in the large intestine was a much more complex problem.

Why the difference? The contents of the small intestine are fluid, consisting of food that is being digested, mixed with digestive juices from the stomach, the liver (bile) and the pancreas, all of which counteract the growth of bacteria. The excrement in the small intestine is therefore still relatively easy to deal with and not overly foul. The small intestine also has an exceptionally good supply of blood and a muscular wall with a strong outer layer of connective tissue. By contrast, the large intestine is packed with bacteria and compact stools, and has a much thinner wall with far fewer blood vessels. There is thus a greater chance of a surgical suture in the large intestine leaking than one in the small intestine, and with much more serious consequences.

In normal circumstances, the risk of a leakage in a large intestine suture is already quite high – around 5 per cent, or one in twenty. But that risk is even greater if the abdomen is infected (peritonitis). There was therefore a very real possibility that this would happen to Karol Wojtyła after the operation, as the contents of his intestines had been leaking into his abdominal cavity for forty-five minutes. The surgical solution to this heightened risk is a stoma, an opening in the abdominal wall, through which the contents of the bowel can be diverted outside the body and no longer pass by the wound in the intestine. This prevents any further leakage.

The use of a stoma emerged out of necessity in the history of surgery. Until the nineteenth century, no one dared to cut open an abdomen. But if one had already been cut open by someone else – by a knife or a sword, for example – it gave the surgeon an opportunity to at least have a try. No one would blame you if the patient died. Theophrastus Bombastus von Hohenheim, one of the most renowned and successful surgeons of the late Middle Ages and better known by his adopted name Paracelsus, was the first to describe placing a stoma on the bowel before the wound as the only way to ensure some hope of the patient's survival. The Latin term for a stoma is '*anus praeternatur-alis*', literally 'beyond-natural anus'. There are various kinds of stomas: they can be temporary (reversible) or permanent (irreversible), be placed on the small intestine (ileostomy) or large intestine (colostomy), and can have one opening (end stoma) or two (double-barrel stoma).

In the case of John Paul II, the safest solution would have been the operation devised by the Frenchman Henri Hartmann in 1921. In what is now known as Hartmann's operation, the affected last section of the large intestine (the sigmoid colon) is removed without connecting the two open ends back together. The lower one is simply closed off and the upper one is used to make a stoma. This makes it a safe operation, as it does not require a suture on the intestine, which might later leak. If the patient's abdomen becomes infected (peritonitis), you can allow that to heal first before joining the intestine together in a second operation. That means that you can wait until the patient and his abdomen are in optimal condition to undergo an operation. The connection in the large intestine then has better chance of healing successfully than in an inflamed abdomen. That is the great benefit of Hartmann's operation – the risk of a leaking suture in the large intestine can be reduced by postponing that part of the operation to a more favourable moment.

The Italian surgeons did something else, however. They stitched up the tear in the large intestine without removing the damaged part and constructed a stoma in the upper section of the large intestine, some half a metre before the tear. The advantage of this option was that it would make the second operation to remove the stoma easier than with Hartmann's operation. It did, however, have the disadvantage that they took a risk by having to leave a large intestine suture behind in an abdominal cavity that contained bacteria.

The operation had been under way for several hours when it was the turn of Crucitti's boss, Giancarlo Castiglione, to storm into the operating room. He was in Milan when he heard the news, had caught a plane to Rome and arrived at the Gemelli Hospital just in time to take over. Castiglione, Crucitti and Salgarello rinsed the pope's abdominal cavity and inserted five drains, silicone or rubber tubes that remove the fluid from the abdomen. They then closed the abdominal wall and took an X-ray, which revealed no bullet. Later, an exit wound was discovered in the pope's buttock and the bullet was found in the popemobile.

After they had also treated the wounds to the index finger and upper arm, five hours and twenty-five minutes had passed. Of course, it was not the real heroes of the hour Salgarello and Crucitti who spoke to the press but their boss, Castiglione. He had a highly developed sense of drama and suggested that the pope's survival had been a miracle, saying, 'If you look at an anatomy book, you cannot find a space wide enough for a bullet to pass through and miss so many vital organs.' That is, of course, nonsense. The pope's anatomy was perfectly normal and the two intestines, which together suffered six holes, and the large bone from which he lost three litres of blood most certainly qualify as vital organs. What he meant was that, if the bullet had passed slightly to one side, it would have hit the major blood vessels. In that case, the delay of three-quarters of an hour between the shot and the operation would have indeed been too long. The pope himself would later help to consolidate this myth. According to Karol Wojtyła, the projectile was guided through his lower abdomen by a 'mother's hand', suggesting the direct intervention of the Virgin Mary.

Five days after the operation, the pope celebrated his sixty-first birthday in the Intensive Care department at the Gemelli Hospital. He went home again on 3 June. But he had developed a cyto-megalovirus infection (CMV) as a result of all the blood transfusions and the wound left by the operation had also become infected. On 20 June, he was readmitted to hospital. Wound infections are not rare after emergency operations in which excrement has entered the abdominal cavity. They often result in the abdominal wall not healing properly, so that much later the scar can rupture to form an incisional hernia, requiring a new operation. This fate would also befall the pope. However, the peritonitis healed quickly and Wojtyła wanted to be rid of the stoma as soon as possible. On 5 August, less than ten weeks after the attack, Crucitti connected the ends of the large intestine back together – a short, 45-minute operation – and, nine days later, the pope was home again.

The popemobile was fitted with a bulletproof cabin. Ağca – who later claimed to be Jesus Christ – spent nineteen years in an Italian jail, where Karol Wojtyła visited him on several occasions. After that, Ağca spent a further ten years in jail in Turkey. He was released in 2010. The blood-smeared white T-shirt made by Swiss underwear manufacturer Hanro that John Paul II had been wearing at the time of the attack was kept as a relic in the chapel of the Daughters of Charity in Rome. The pope rewarded Salgarello and his colleagues by investing them with the Order of St Gregory the Great, the highest honour bestowed by the Vatican.

A year later, there was a second attack on John Paul II. A disturbed Spanish priest wounded him superficially with a bayonet. After spending three years in prison the priest, Juan María Fernández y Krohn, set up a lawyer's practice in Belgium.

From 1984, Karol Wojtyła was regularly to be found skiing incognito in the mountains of Abruzzo. But in 1991, his health started to deteriorate. He developed Parkinson's disease and, in 1992, was diagnosed with a precancerous polyp in the large intestine. The tumour was discovered in the sigmoid colon, precisely the part of the large intestine that Ağca's bullet had passed through. It is not very probable that the one had anything to do with the other, but if the surgeons had conducted Hartmann's operation back in 1981 and had removed the torn

Surgical team

During an operation, a modern operating room is strictly divided between a sterile (clean and completely bacteria-free) and a non-sterile (clean, but not completely bacteria-free) field. The part of the patient to be operated on is cleaned with disinfectant. The rest of the patient is covered with sterilised paper drapes. Everyone in the operating room wears clean surgical scrubs, cap and mask. The operation is performed by the surgeon and an assisting surgeon. They are aided by the scrub nurse, a surgical assistant who is responsible for the instruments and other materials used. These three people are 'sterile' – they wear gowns and gloves that have been sterilised and are completely free of bacteria. They have to ensure they remain sterile by not touching anything outside the sterile field. All instruments and other materials, such as sutures for stitching, have also been sterilised and may only be touched by these three people. A second surgical assistant – known as the circulating nurse or surgical technologist – is not dressed in sterile clothing and supplies the materials to the operating team in a way that ensures they remain sterile. An important job for the circulating assistant is to count the gauzes used during the operation. At the head end of the operating table is the anaesthetist, the doctor who administers the anaesthetic, with an assistant. Six people are thus needed for each patient, three of whom are dressed in sterile clothing (in the past, too, surgeons could not perform operations alone – they needed four assistants to hold on to the patient's arms and legs).

section of the large intestine, then a tumour could not have developed there. Now the old man's sigmoid colon was removed after all, and he recovered from this operation reasonably well, too. The operation was carried out by one of the same surgeons as eleven years previously, Francesco Crucitti. During the operation, the pope's gall bladder was also removed to alleviate a problem with gallstones.

In 1993, Karol Wojtyła fell down the stairs, dislocating his shoulder. In 1994, he slipped in the bathroom and broke his hip. He was operated on and given an artificial hip. In 1995, a third attack was planned on the pope, by Al Qaeda in the Philippines, but it was foiled in time. In 1996, he was operated on for a dubious case of appendicitis.

Pope John Paul II lived to be an old man, but kept his sense of humour. When, shortly after his hip operation, he rose from his stool with considerable difficulty, drawn with pain and stiff as a board, he mischievously and brilliantly quoted Galileo Galilei, mumbling '*Eppure, si muove!*' – and yet it moves!

The deterioration of the aged pope was painfully and graphically reported in the media. In 2005, the now demented old man was given a tracheotomy, a breathing tube in the neck, because he was having difficulties with coughing. A month later, he died of an infection in the urinary tract. He had undoubtedly undergone more operations than any other pope in history. He was canonised in 2014.

He donated the bullet that had pierced his abdomen – and was supposedly guided safely past his major blood vessels by the hand of the Virgin Mary – to Our Lady of Fátima in Portugal, out of gratitude for this fortuitous intervention. It can be seen there in the crown worn by the statue, hanging above her head like a sword of Damocles.

7

Fracture

Dr Democedes and the Greek Method: King Darius

I N ONE OF the most exciting books of all time, *The Histories*
– written more than 2,400 years ago – Herodotus tells a story
that was then already a century old. It is about a man who,
at the age of about thirty-three, fell from his horse while hunting
and dislocated his ankle, leaving his foot incorrectly positioned
below his leg.

Little is said about the circumstances of the accident, but much
about what followed. A doctor pulled the foot back into place.
In medical terms, that is known as reposition. That caused the
man so much pain, however, that he asked another doctor for a
second opinion. The latter's advice was clear and simple – rest.
Apparently the ankle recovered fully, as he conducted one military campaign after the other until he was finally defeated during
a battle near Marathon in Greece. He was none other than Darius
the Great, King of Persia, builder of the world's very first asphalted
highway and founder of the city of Persepolis. He called himself
'the King of Kings'.

The first doctor – the one who had caused him so much pain
– was an Egyptian physician in service to the king. At that time,
Egyptians were considered the best doctors. In actual fact, there
was nothing wrong with his treatment, despite Darius not being
satisfied with it. It would have been a big mistake not to pull
the crooked ankle back straight again. A displaced foot has to be
realigned with the the lower leg as soon as possible. Until that

happens, the foot receives too little blood and starts to die off. But you needed guts to pull on the dislocated ankle of Darius. After all, as a doctor in Persia you had to comply with the thousand-year-old laws of King Hammurabi of Babylon. Known as the Code of Hammurabi, they have been preserved for posterity on a large pillar of black basalt more than two metres high, which can now be seen in the Louvre in Paris.

The code was based on the rules of trade and surgeons would enter into an agreement with their clients: if the treatment was successful, they were paid. If not, they received nothing. If it went wrong, they were called to account – an eye for an eye, a tooth for a tooth – just like everyone else. Article 197 of the code states that if a man should break the bone of another, one of his bones should also be broken – unless the bone in question belonged to a slave. Then, under article 199, it was sufficient to pay half the value of the slave or – under article 198 – one gold mina if it were a freed slave. Article 218 says that if a patient died at the hands of a surgeon, the surgeon's own hands were to be cut off. It may have been less lucrative to treat slaves, but it was much safer; under article 219, if a slave died during treatment, you could replace him with a slave of equal value – and keep your hands.

The code has nothing to say about the doctor–patient relationship in the case of kings. Article 202 does state that a man who strikes someone of a higher rank or status shall receive sixty strokes with an oxtail whip in public. King Darius was, of course, above the law. He was so enraged by the pain from his foot that he ordered all his Egyptian physicians to be crucified.

The second doctor who told Darius to rest was none other than Democedes of Croton, famed throughout Greece but at the time a prisoner of Darius. Democedes had been personal physician to Polycrates, the ruler of Samos, but had been captured along with the entourage of Polycrates. He was not noticed until Darius urgently needed a doctor for a second opinion.

According to Herodotus, Democedes treated Darius's ankle the Greek way, meaning 'with a gentle hand'. The historian speaks as though Democedes knew exactly what he was doing, while all the other (non-Greek) doctors did not. His method must have been a great success, as Darius recovered completely and showered him with gifts and he was appointed as a slave to the Persian court. It is likely however, that Democedes did little more than examine the patient and conclude that the foot (thanks to his Egyptian colleague) was sufficiently straight and vital. All he had to do was reassure the king and prescribe him rest – that is to say, to be patient – and let the healing power of the body work its magic. Sometimes good care is that simple.

Except, of course, that the story is most likely untrue. Herodotus had every reason to boast about the Greeks and their healing skills. He was himself a Greek and, at the time he wrote this story about the Greek slave who had saved the Persian king, Athens had just been destroyed by the Persians in the Second Persian War. Darius had begun the First Persian War, but was defeated at the Battle of Marathon in 490 AD. His son Xerxes then started a second campaign against Greece and, although it was the greatest military campaign ever seen in history, the Greeks again refused to succumb. Herodotus did his utmost to remain as objective as possible about the Persians but, nevertheless, this story about Darius's ankle must be interpreted as Greek propaganda in the aftermath of the two Persian wars. With today's surgical knowledge, it is difficult to believe that the dislocated ankle of such an important historic figure could have left no traces in records. And to heal an ankle joint without a lasting functional impairment or chronic pain calls for a precision that cannot have been possible in those times.

The ankle is comprised of the *talus*, the uppermost bone in the foot, which fits neatly as a tenon into the ankle mortise of the lower leg. The ankle mortise is a rectangular socket of bones, formed on the inner and upper side by the *tibia* (shinbone) and on the outer side by the *fibula* (the calf bone). The foot fits into this structure so snugly that, in the event of a trauma to the ankle, it can only move out of position if the bones of the ankle mortise break. If the broken bones are then not replaced in exactly the same place – to the millimetre – and the talus therefore no longer hinges precisely in the ankle mortise, this will cause wear and tear, leading to degenerative joint disease. That is especially problematic in the ankle, as the joint bears the full weight of the body with every step and the forces are even greater when running and jumping. Severe fractures of the ankle joint are therefore notorious for leading to chronic functional impairment, pain and disability. None of these appear to have occurred in the case of King Darius.

A precise repositioning of the fractured bones, in such a way that the ankle joint is exactly restored, only really became possible with the invention of the plaster cast in 1851, by Dutch army surgeon Antonius Mathijsen, the discovery of X-rays by Wilhelm Conrad Röntgen in 1895, and the development of a completely new operational technique by the Arbeitsgemeinschaft für Osteosynthesefragen (AO Foundation) in Switzerland in 1958. Today, the treatment almost always involves an operation whereby, using X-rays, the broken pieces are held firmly in place with metal plates and screws. This method is known as osteosynthesis, literally 'joining the bone together'. It is usually a very fiddly job getting all the small pieces of bone to fit back together exactly and then fixing them with screws. In the case of an ankle, this can take a good hour, from the first incision to the final stitch.

If Darius's ankle was not broken, is it possible that his foot could have been displaced without a fracture to the ankle fork? He would then have suffered a luxation of the joint, more commonly referred to as a dislocation. A pure dislocation of the ankle is extremely rare and requires exceptionally strong bones. We can assume, however

Traumatology, surgery and orthopaedics

Traumatology – the treatment of injuries and wounds caused by accidents – is a typical surgical activity. It becomes very important in war. A good army surgeon was worth his weight in gold to a king, as a patched-up soldier can fight again. In peacetime, traumatology was fuelled by crime, and traffic and accidents at work. Fixing fractures and caring for gaping wounds was the job of the surgeon, who 'healed' – that is, made things whole again. For a long time, in peacetime, traumatology was performed by barbers. They happened to have a perfect treatment chair, a wash basin and a clean blade to hand. After a successful operation, the barber would hang the blood-spattered white bandages outside on a stick, as a sign of his trade. This is the origin of the red-and-white stick you still see hanging outside barber's shops today. Orthopaedics originally had nothing to do with surgery and did not involve the use of knives, blades or scalpels. The word comes from the Greek *orthos*, meaning straight, and *paidion* (child), and the focus lay on fitting children with braces and splints to correct deformities of the bones. Today orthopaedists treat all kinds of abnormalities of the bones and joints, not only among children and no longer without using a scalpel. With the advent of joint replacement surgery, orthopaedics has become a fully fledged surgical discipline.

that Darius did not have strong bones, a conclusion that can be drawn from a scientific experiment conducted by Herodotus himself – without him being aware of it.

The historian had been to Egypt as a tourist and had visited the site in the desert where the first battle had taken place between the Persians, led by King Cambyses, Darius's mad predecessor, and the Egyptians, under the leadership of Pharaoh Psamtik. The Persians had won, but only after severe losses on both sides. As was customary, after the battle (or rather, the slaughter), the bodies had been separated and piled up. Herodotus had stood and looked at the piles of skeletons and, in a sudden fit of touristic vandalism, threw rocks at them. He observed that it was possible to make a hole in the skulls of the Persians with only a small stone, while those of the Egyptians refused to break even if you hammered away at them with a sizeable rock. Herodotus attributed the difference to the sun, which shone down on the heads of the bare-headed Egyptians for their whole lives, while the Persians always wore felt hats or carried parasols (you do indeed get strong bones from the sun, but not for the reason Herodotus thought – it comes from the vitamin D engendered by sunlight).

If we could examine Darius's skeleton, we could measure the strength of his bones. We might even be able to find traces of a fractured ankle, if he had one. Just as a wound in the skin always leaves a scar, a wound to a bone – in other words, a fracture – also leaves its traces many years later, at least in adults. That is because bone, like skin, is living tissue.

Bone consists of cells supplied with blood by small blood vessels that criss-cross the thick calcium layers. That is why, if a bone breaks, it will bleed. The calcium, however, gets in the way of the healing process. That problem is solved by osteoclasts (literally, 'bone-demolishers'), special cells that clear the area around the wound by eating away a few millimetres of bone tissue on either side of the fracture. After the osteoclasts have done their work, it is the turn of the osteoblasts ('bone builders'), cells that produce connective tissue to fill the gap. Because this is a process that takes up more space than the gap allows, a lump is created at the site of the fracture. This lump, known as a callus, contains young bone cells called osteocytes, which deposit calcium, so that the fresh callus becomes stronger. It takes around two months for the callus to bridge the fracture sufficiently. The young bone then gradually matures until there is eventually no difference in structure from the rest of the bone. But the callus remains as a scar.

Unfortunately, we cannot conduct a post-mortem on Darius to see if there is a callus on his ankle. The Persians did adopt the practice of mummification from the Egyptians but, although Darius's tomb has been found, hewn out of a rock in Naqš-e-Rostām in present-day Iran, his mummy is no longer in it. Exactly what happened to his foot during the hunt that day will forever remain a mystery.

What does Herodotus tell us about the fate of Democedes? He proved not only to have a 'gentle hand' but also to be a gentle man, showing great solidarity with his Egyptian colleagues, as he persuaded Darius to spare their lives. He suffered terribly from homesickness and was afraid that he would never return to Greece now the king was so pleased with him. But when Queen Atossa developed an abscess in her breast and Democedes successfully cut it open, he asked the king to reward him by allowing him to return to Greece. Darius made him part of a spying mission to prepare for the imminent invasion of Greece. He was to serve as guide and interpreter for a group of scouts. Democedes, however, took advantage of the opportunity to escape. Back in his birthplace of Croton, he married the daughter of Milon the wrestler. So ended a brilliant career that had started in Aegina, where he was paid 60 mina (1 talent) a year in the service of the state. He later received 100 mina in Athens and a year later 120 as physician to Polycrates on Samos – a salary that roughly corresponds to that of a modern surgeon, if you take the price of bread then and now for comparison. Due to an unfortunate change of course in his career he found himself working for Darius the Great. Although he was the most famous doctor of his time, in the history books he would be completely overshadowed by another Greek doctor, who also spoke of the gentle hand and of solidarity among colleagues: Hippocrates.

And of course the Code of Hammurabi has failed to withstand the ravages of time. Hammurabi had warned that anyone who changed his laws would be inflicted with 'high fever and severe wounds that cannot be healed' by the goddess Nin-karak and struck down by the inexorable curse of the supreme god Bel. Despite the warning, the duty to provide a result ('no cure, no pay') was replaced. In modern medical law, the patient is no longer a client who buys a product. That has been changed to a duty to provide a best effort ('duty of care'). Surgeons no longer commit themselves to achieve a result but to do their best to achieve it. This protects the surgeon, because sometimes the result may not be possible. In the case of harm, too, the onus of guilt is shifted from the result to the intention: surgeons who do their best to prevent harm cannot be called to account for any harm caused.

This distinction between anyone who harms another with a knife and a surgeon who treats someone using a scalpel has been laid down in modern law. The concepts of competence and authority determine who is guilty and who is not. A qualified surgeon is authorised but, as long as he practises his profession, he must ensure that his competence remains up to scratch, by accumulating experience, taking refresher courses, and achieving good results.

8

Varicose Veins

Lucy and Modern-Day Surgery: *Australopithecus afarensis*

O UR BODIES ARE made up of components that, after billions of years of trial and error, have become closely related to each other at macroscopic, cellular and molecular level. To understand them, you need knowledge of several natural sciences, including biology, biochemistry and genetics. They are so complex that it is easy to overlook the fact that many of those components work surprisingly simply. The venous valves in our veins, which prevent the blood from flowing in the reverse direction, are a good example. The explanation of how they work may seem a little technical, but with some knowledge of gravity and pressure, they are easy to understand.

On the inside of each of our legs, a long vein runs just below the skin, from the ankle right up to the groin. This is the great saphenous vein, or GSV for short (one origin of the word 'saphenous' is *saphon*, the Latin for 'cable'). Together with a number of smaller veins, the GSV comes out in the groin in a short, curved section of vein resembling a shepherd's crook, called the saphenous arch. In the saphenous arch, there is a small valve. This is nothing out of the ordinary, as all veins below this point have valves, to stop the blood from flowing back downwards under the influence of gravity. Strangely enough, however, there is not a single valve to be found in the long stretch of veins above the saphenous arch, from the groin to the heart. In an adult human, during the day, that one small valve in the saphenous arch therefore has to resist the pressure of a column of liquid some 50 centimetres long. That is five times greater than the pressure on any of the other valves in our veins. A lot to expect from a valve that is otherwise completely normal, not especially strong or built to withstand such high pressure. As a result, the small valve in the saphenous arch can sometimes malfunction. It no longer stops the backflow of blood and starts to 'leak'. This can cause varicose veins.

Varicose veins are abnormally enlarged subcutaneous veins through which the blood flows upwards too slowly, does not flow at all, or even flows back downwards. They are not only unsightly, but can also cause problems, such as pain, itching and eczema in the surrounding skin. They usually start with a leaking valve, often the valve in the saphenous arch, as that is most under pressure. If the valve fails, the pressure is relocated downwards to the following valve, around ten centimetres lower down the leg. This valve then has to cope with the column of liquid, which is now ten centimetres longer. If that valve also fails, there is even more pressure on the next one. In this way, the pressure steadily rises and the GSV will gradually blow up like an elongated balloon. Eventually, all the valves will leak and the GSV, normally no thicker than half a centimetre, will enlarge to form varicose veins, which can in some places grow to the size of a bunch of grapes.

So the cause for varicose veins is that one small valve in the saphenous arch is too weak for the job it is supposed to do because, for some mysterious reason, there are no valves in the large veins above it. The obvious question is: why? The answer is staggeringly simple.

To find it, we have to go back 3.2 million years, to Lucy, a twenty-five-year-old *Australopithecus afarensis*. Lucy and the other members of her species were among the first of our ancestors to walk on two legs. Lucy, by walking upright, is at the root of half of modern-day surgical practice. Parts of her skeleton were found in Ethiopia in 1974 by paleoanthropologists Donald Johanson and

Tom Gray. They called her after the Beatles' song 'Lucy in the Sky with Diamonds', which was playing on the radio when they were digging. Lucy is currently to be seen in the national museum in Addis Ababa and replicas can be found in museums all around the world.

Let us assume that Lucy's mother still walked on all four legs. That meant that the liquid column in the major veins between her groin and heart was horizontal. And because no pressure builds up in a horizontal liquid column, Lucy's ancestors did not suffer from varicose veins. Valves in the major veins 'above' the saphenous arch would have been pointless for the simple reason that they were not above it.

Varicose veins are therefore as old as the modern human. The first report of varicose veins is from Egypt and is more than 3,500 years old. The earliest illustration dates from the golden age of Athens, and Hippocrates was the first to treat them with bandages. The Roman Celsus described the removing of varicose veins by making an incision and drawing them out with a blunt hook. According to Plutarch, consul Gaius Marius, the uncle of Julius Caesar, was more affected by the pain of this operation than by the result, and refused to allow his second leg to be operated on. Pliny tells us that this tough-guy statesman was the only one to undergo the operation standing up, refusing to be bound to the operating table. Tough indeed, but also a little foolish as, because of the higher pressure in the vertical liquid column, much more blood spurts out of the open varicose veins during the operation than if the patient is lying down.

The valves in the veins were not described until after the Middle Ages. Even so, that does not mean they were understood. Ambroise Paré was the first surgeon to think of tying off the GSV with a ligature high in the upper leg. We now know that doing this cannot cause any real harm, as there are plenty of veins to take over the work of the GSV – but did Paré know that?

In 1890, German surgeon Friedrich Trendelenburg described the high ligature in greater detail and was the first to display some insight into varicose veins being caused by the leaking of the venous valves and the increased hydraulic pressure. This marked the step to functional treatment. The position of the patient on their back, with the operating table tilted with the head down and the feet up, is named after him. In the Trendelenburg position, the hydraulic pressure is reversed, becoming negative in the legs and positive in the heart. The increase in pressure in the heart is favourable for patients in shock and the low pressure in the legs is better for performing varicose vein operations.

At the end of the nineteenth century, Australian surgeon Jerry Moore perfected the methods of Paré and Trendelenburg. He understood that you should not tie off the GSV as high as possible, but go one step further and tie off the saphenous arch. This became the standard method in modern times, and is known as a crossectomy, after the French for a shepherd's crook, *crosse*. The procedure not only allows the existing, visible varicose veins to be treated, but also prevents the problem from reoccurring.

In the twentieth century, the crossectomy was combined with 'stripping', a method by which the GSV can be removed subcutaneously completely and in one go. This was – and remained until around 2005 – the standard procedure for treating varicose veins, the whole operation taking no more than fifteen minutes per leg. Theodor Billroth, one of the greatest names in the whole history of surgery, was vehemently opposed to varicose vein operations, without bothering to explain why.

And then came Sven Ivar Seldinger, a Swedish radiologist who turned the whole of vascular surgery on its head. In 1953, he invented a method that made it possible to treat blood vessels endovascularly – from the inside. Thanks to the Seldinger method, in 1964 another radiologist called Charles Dotter invented percutaneous angioplasty,

Circulation

The heart consists of two halves. The right half pumps blood from the body to the lungs under slight pressure. The lungs are delicate and cannot withstand high pressures. The left half of the heart pumps the blood from the lungs to the rest of the body. Here, the blood pressure is much higher. Arteries transport the oxygen-rich, bright-red blood from the heart to the furthest edges of the body. Veins collect the blood from the whole body and carry it back to the heart. The workings of the heart and the blood vessels – the circulation – was a complete mystery until 1628, when the Englishman William Harvey spent several hours looking at the beating heart of a dying deer, which he had cut open while it was still alive. He described his findings in a treatise entitled *Exercitatio Anatomica the Motu Cordis et Sanguinis in Animalibus*. No one had ever understood the body's circulatory system before mainly because, after death, blood coagulates, so that the blood vessels of a corpse seem to mainly contain air. The return of the blood to the heart occurs through a combination of the movement of the limbs and the valves in the veins. This is known as the skeletal-muscle pump. The suction power of the chest also helps this process. When we breathe in, negative pressure is created in the chest cavity, drawing blood up out of the abdomen and the limbs. The veins of the digestive system and the spleen are an exception in the circulation system. Known as portal veins, they transport the blood to the liver, rather than back to the heart.

a brilliantly simple idea for the treatment of narrowed arteries by stretching the blood vessel from the inside with a small balloon. In the twenty-first century, the Seldinger method is used to treat not only arteries, but also varicose veins. The GSV can be seared from the inside with laser or microwave treatment to seal it off. And all without the need for a scalpel.

Lucy brought humankind even more problems. If she did not happen to have three small blood vessels in her rectum that kept her anus watertight (the haemorrhoidal veins), she would probably have changed her mind after her first few steps and gone back to walking on four legs. The act of defecation has never succeeded in adapting: we still have to bend our hips at 90 degrees to do it. The fact that this now requires much greater pressure leads to typical human problems like haemorrhoids, prolapses and constipation.

Another regular feature in the daily work of a surgeon that we have Lucy to thank for is the inguinal canal. This is a weak spot at the bottom of the abdominal wall, exactly where it should be at its strongest. Gravity continually forces the contents of the abdomen against the inside of this weak spot. That can lead to a hole, known as an inguinal or groin hernia, an opening that evolution seems to have forgotten. But if we imagine ourselves on four legs again, the inguinal canal then appears to be higher than the centre of gravity of the abdomen, not lower. So no problem for our four-legged friends, but a real design flaw for us bipeds. Because we walk upright, modern men have a 25 per cent chance of developing a groin hernia in their lifetimes. And that means plenty of work for the surgeon.

The transition from quadruped to biped also meant of course that the hips and knees had to bear twice as much weight. And the intervertebral discs, which separate the individual vertebrae in the spine, went from supporting practically nothing (horizontally) to carrying half the body weight (vertically). This excessive load on the knees, hips and back led to the development of a sister discipline of surgery – orthopaedics. Orthopaedic surgeons spend a large part of their time replacing overburdened hips and knees with prostheses and removing hernias in the back.

The most conspicuous fault can be seen in the arteries running to the legs. They still make a 90-degree bend characteristic of quadrupeds, deep down at the back of the pelvis. This bend was necessary because the hind legs of an animal are at right angles to the trunk. Since we spent most of the time we were evolving from primitive land animals to humans walking on four legs, natural selection has made the 90-degree bend in our arteries wide, spacious and gradual. That causes the least possible turbulence in this stretch of the circulation system, which is important for our survival, as turbulence in the arteries can cause damage to the artery wall. Because we now walk upright, however, after making the gentle, gradual bend of the quadruped, the leg arteries now have to bend back another 90-degrees in the groin. This is not a smooth curve, but a sharp kink that has not adapted and does cause turbulence. That leads to hardening of the arteries (arteriosclerosis), resulting in narrowing of the blood vessels near the kink. And that is why hardening of the arteries in humans is most common in the groin. If the arteries gradually become narrower, the legs receive insufficient oxygen-rich blood at the moment that they need it most – during exercise. That causes pain when walking, which disappears immediately again when standing still. This condition is known medically as intermittent claudication (from the Latin *claudicare*, 'to limp'), but in Dutch it is appropriately called 'window-shopping legs', referring to the fact that the pain of walking down the street will subside every time you stop to look in a shop window. Eventually, the legs can die off, causing gangrene. This is not something quadrupeds have to worry about.

And so we have accumulated quite a list of complaints treated by modern-day surgeons that can be traced back to Lucy. Varicose veins, haemorrhoids, groin hernias and narrowing of the arteries account for perhaps half the work of the average surgical practice. In other words, a large part of the work of the surgeon consists of patching up what went wrong when Lucy decided to walk on two legs. Incidentally, Lucy was given a second name, in Ethiopian – *Dinqines*, which means 'you are amazing'. Surgeons can agree with that.

9

Peritonitis

The Death of an Escape Artist: Harry Houdini

WHEN ERIK WEISZ died on 31 October 1926, it was world news. On this side of the Atlantic, it was a time of guarded optimism. But there was also poverty and unrest, and two as yet unknown men called Adolf Hitler and Benito Mussolini were preparing themselves for a leading role in global politics. It was the year Claude Monet died and Marilyn Monroe was born. Europe looked jealously at America, where everything seemed possible and where these years – until the Great Crash of 1929 – were known as the Roaring Twenties. It was the era of the Charleston and Prohibition, of Rockefeller and Al Capone.

Like Charlie Chaplin, Stan Laurel and Oliver Hardy, Erik Weisz typified the spirit of that wonderful time in America. Almost no one knew his real name but his stage name is still – almost a century later – known around the world and has become synonymous with the art that he developed. Erik Weisz was the world-famous Harry Houdini, the escape artist who had himself buttoned up into a straitjacket and hoisted up in the air by his feet, wrapped in chains and sealed in a wooden chest and then thrown overboard in New York harbour, handcuffed and shut in a milk churn full of beer. And he always emerged unharmed, even after being buried alive in a bronze coffin. Many will think that his death was as spectacular as his life, that he drowned while performing his legendary Chinese Water Torture

Cell act – handcuffed, upside down and underwater, on stage, in front of a packed theatre. But nothing is further from the truth.

Houdini ornamented his spectacular escape acts with Spiritism and classical circus tricks. He was a juggler, an acrobat and a strong-man. He claimed, for example, that his abdominal muscles could withstand any blow and challenged everyone to try it out. For a long time, it was assumed that his death had been caused by one of these hefty punches in his stomach, but we know now that it had nothing to do with his stunts and was largely down to his stubborn refusal to go to a doctor.

Gordon Whitehead, Jacques Price and Sam Smilovitz were three Canadian students. They visited Houdini in his dressing room in the theatre in Montreal on 22 October 1926, the morning after his performance. Houdini lay on a divan to pose for Smilovitz, who wanted to draw a portrait of him. Whitehead asked him if it was true that he could withstand any blow to his stomach and whether he could give it a try. Houdini agreed and the student immediately started to punch him. He hit Houdini several times extremely hard in his right lower abdomen. The two other young men later stated that the escape artist was clearly not ready for their friend's rapid attack. They saw that he had only been able to tense his abdominal muscles sufficiently after the third blow and they noticed that, as the tough escape artist – who had been so magnificently indestructible on the stage the previous night – lay there on the divan, he seemed to be suffering unexpected terrible pain from the few well-aimed punches.

Houdini left the following day, after his evening show, taking the train to Detroit, the next stop on his tour. He was not feeling well and sent a telegram ahead asking to see a doctor when he arrived. But once he got to the city, he had no time to be examined and started the final performance of his life with a high fever. He may have performed his underwater escape act, which entailed him holding his breath for several minutes – a fantastic achievement considering that, after the show, a doctor had no hesitation in concluding that he needed to be operated on immediately. The audience thus had no idea just what an incredible stuntman they were watching up there on the stage.

The surgeon at the hospital in Detroit made his diagnosis with a simple physical examination. Laying his hand on Houdini's abdomen, he declared that the escape artist was suffering from an everyday complaint – appendicitis – but which was only just then starting to be understood. It had only been correctly described for the first time forty years earlier (when Houdini was twelve years old) by Reginald Fitz in Boston. That is remarkable for a life-threatening illness that must have been affecting people for thousands of years. There is no mention of it in ancient Mesopotamian, Egyptian, Greek or Roman medical texts, while it must have been prevalent in these old civilisations, where knowledge of medicine was already quite advanced. It was first described by Giovanni Battista Morgagni, an eighteenth-century anatomist, but he too was unable to put his finger on the correct cause of its lethal consequences. Only in 1887 did it become clear that this illness did not have to end in the death of the patient, when Dr Thomas Morton in Philadelphia conducted the first successful operation to treat it.

Houdini should therefore have simply gone to hospital in Montreal, where he could have been saved by an operation. Was he too stubborn, too vain, too money-driven, or simply afraid of doctors? He probably thought 'the show must go on'. Consequently, he was not operated on until three days later in Detroit. The surgeon discovered peritonitis, which develops from the bursting of the appendix. Houdini's abdominal cavity was completely infected with pus. Four days later his abdomen had to be opened up again to be rinsed out. But the situation did not improve and there were at that time no antibiotics to fight the infection.

Medical terms

Medical complaints and diseases are indicated by words ending in *-osis*. Arthrosis is therefore a complaint affecting a joint (*arthron*) (caused by wear and tear). Words ending in *-itis* indicate an inflammation: arthritis is an inflamed joint. Not all inflammations are infections. They are only referred to as infections if they are caused by propagating pathogens, such as bacteria, viruses and other parasites. The prefix *a* or *an* means 'without' and *ec* or *ex* mean 'out'. Apnoea means 'without breathing' and a tumourectomy means cutting out a tumour. Haem(at)o is related to blood. Haematuria is blood in the urine, haemoptysis is the act of coughing up blood. A tumour (Latin for 'swelling') is indicated by the ending *-oma*. It can be an accumulation of fluid; a haematoma, for example, is a collection of blood. But tumours can also be made of solid tissue. A lipoma is a tumour consisting of fatty tissue. Tumours can be malignant or benign. Malignant tumours are cancerous and their names end with carcinoma (cancer of the skin, mucous membrane or gland tissue) or sarcoma (cancer of other tissues, such as bone or muscle). Benign tumours are not cancerous. The result of a test is positive if it confirms the diagnosis or if it reveals a disorder. A positive result is therefore often negative for a patient. Furthermore, no tests are 100 per cent reliable. A result can thus sometimes be falsely positive or negative. The ending *-genic* indicates a cause. If something is carcinogenic, it can give you cancer.

Harry Houdini died two days later, at the age of fifty-two. He was buried in Queens, New York, amid a whirl of public attention, in the same bronze coffin he had used for his escape acts. Erik Weisz, juggler, stuntman, Spiritist and, above all, escape artist – known around the world as The Great Houdini – died of a banal, everyday complaint: appendicitis.

Appendicitis is a very common disease. More than 8 per cent of men and almost 7 per cent of women contract appendicitis at some time in their lives. It can occur at any age and is the most common cause of acute abdominal pain. The appendix – more correctly the vermiform ('worm-shaped') appendix – is a blind-ended intestinal tube starting from the great bowel near the junction with the small bowel, located in the right lower quadrant of the abdomen. It is less than a centimetre in diameter and some ten centimetres long.

Doctors knew about the small organ for a long time, but it had never occurred to anyone that such a small thing could have such disastrous consequences. It is because it is so small that, once it is inflamed, it can burst quite quickly. The contents of the intestines are then released into the abdomen, which causes peritonitis, inflammation of the entire peritoneum, the lining of the abdominal cavity. And that is why the link was never made between that small appendix and the fatal consequences of an abdominal inflammation. Before surgeons dared to open up a living patient's abdomen with any degree of success in the nineteenth century, they only saw the final state of the appendix in the body of the deceased. During the autopsy, amid the debris of full-scale peritonitis, no one had ever noticed the rupture of that tiny, worm-shaped appendage.

Appendicitis generates a typical series of symptoms that reflect the successive stages of the disease, starting with the inflammation of the appendix itself. This causes a vague organic pain in the centre of the upper abdomen. Within a day, the inflammation expands around the appendix and starts to irritate the peritoneum in the area where it is located, on the right side of the lower abdomen. This local pain is much more acute and pronounced than the vague organic pain. Typically, patients with appendicitis describe the pain as moving downwards from the centre to the lower right of the abdomen, increasing in severity as it does so.

The local irritation of the peritoneum also causes fever, loss of appetite (anorexia) and, above all, pain during movement. Patients can no longer tolerate being touched or making sudden movements, and prefer to lie still, flat on their backs with their legs pulled up. For a normal person in this stage of the disease, it would seem impossible to remain standing in front of a theatre full of people, not to mention allow themselves to be tied up, hung upside down and immersed in the Chinese Water Torture Cell as Houdini did.

Pus then forms around the appendix. At first, the pus can be contained by the surrounding intestines, but in the next stage the appendix dies off locally and bursts. Faeces and intestinal gases are then released into the abdominal cavity. The patient experiences a sudden increase in the pain in the lower right of the abdomen, which then spreads throughout the whole abdomen and becomes so severe that it is no longer possible to say exactly where it is coming from. This is the stage of life-threatening peritonitis.

The total picture that fits in with peritonitis is typically that of an 'irritated abdomen'. The abdominal muscles are tense, the abdomen is hard and every movement is painful. It is not only painful when the abdomen is touched, but even more so when it is released – this is known as 'rebound tenderness'. The patient's face is pale, anxious and tense, with sunken eyes and cheeks. The intestines in the abdomen respond to the inflammation by stopping their normal movements. Through a stethoscope, the abdomen is unnaturally quiet. All of these symptoms are so typical of peritonitis that it can be diagnosed in a couple of seconds, with a quick look at the patient (face and position), a few questions (where does it hurt and where and when did it start?), pressing the abdomen once (hard and painful when pressure is applied and released) and listening with the stethoscope (no audible intestinal movements). In the final stage, the patient experiences septic shock caused by blood poisoning; the peritoneum has a large surface area, allowing a mass release of bacteria into the bloodstream. That leads to general poisoning of the body, causing high fever and affecting all organs, with death as the result.

Peritonitis is an acute surgical emergency. The surgeon has to repair or remove the cause as soon as possible and rinse the abdominal cavity. This should be done at the earliest stage possible, preferably before the onset of septic shock or, even better, before the stage of general peritonitis, but the best time is while the problem is still restricted to the affected organ, the tiny appendix. Acute appendicitis is therefore already a surgical emergency.

In 1889, American surgeon Charles McBurney described these principles for operating on appendicitis, namely the sooner the operation is performed, the greater the chances of a full recovery, and that it is sufficient to remove the inflamed organ as long as peritonitis has not yet developed. This linked McBurney irrevocably to appendicitis. The spot on the abdomen where the most pain usually occurs is known as McBurney's point and the incision in the abdominal wall to perform the appendectomy is also named after him. Every surgeon knows immediately what the problem is if a colleague says that a patient has 'tenderness at McBurney's point'.

A classical operation for appendicitis proceeds as follows. The patient lies on his back, the surgeon standing to his right and the assistant to the left. The surgeon makes a small, diagonal incision in the lower right of the abdomen, at McBurney's point, which is exactly two-thirds of the way down an imaginary line between the navel and the bony projection of the iliac crest, the outer edge of the pelvis. There, beneath the skin and the subcutaneous tissue, are three abdominal muscles on top of each other. At exactly this point in the abdominal wall, these muscles can be passed without cutting them, by manoeuvring between the muscle fibres, as though you are opening three pairs of curtains. Below the third muscle is the peritoneum. You have to take hold of this carefully and open it up, making sure you do not damage the intestines. If you are lucky, you can now see the appendix but, usually, it is hidden away somewhere in the depths of the abdomen. You can feel around for it with your finger, free it carefully and pull it outwards. Using a small clamp and an absorbable thread, you first divide and tie off the blood vessel feeding the appendix. You then do the same with the appendix itself. You can now close the peritoneum, move the muscles back in place, and close the aponeurosis, the flat tendon of the outermost of the three abdominal muscles. Lastly, you close the subcutaneous tissue and the skin. The whole business takes about twenty minutes. Today, however, the appendix is no longer removed using the classical procedure. Now, a laparoscopic appendectomy is preferred, using keyhole surgery via the navel and two very small incisions.

Houdini's symptoms were typical of appendicitis – fever and pain in the lower right of the abdomen. The doctor who was only permitted to examine him in his dressing room in Detroit after the show encountered a seriously sick man with an irritated lower right abdomen. The symptoms were so obvious that the doctors did not even consider the punch in the stomach that Gordon Whitehead had given Houdini three days previously. The diagnosis was confirmed during the operation – they found a perforated appendix and the consequential peritonitis. And yet, it was the punches to the stomach that were the focus of attention later. Other cases of alleged 'traumatic appendicitis' – that is, caused by a direct blow, fall or other trauma to the abdomen – were cited. No causal link has, however, ever been found between trauma and appendicitis, and the fact that these two events occurred within days of each other must be seen as coincidence. Nevertheless, the cause of appendicitis is by no means always clear. We do not know why some people contract appendicitis at a certain moment, while others never do.

In the case of Houdini, it was apparently important to find a cause. The three students were extensively interrogated by the police and the punch delivered by poor Gordon Whitehead was established as the clear cause of death. It may have also been significant that Houdini, given his not entirely danger-free profession, had taken out life insurance that included an accident clause. The clause stated that his wife and lifelong assistant Bess Weisz would receive a double pay-out – 500,000 dollars – if Houdini died as the result of an accident while performing a stunt. While a punch in the stomach to demonstrate his strength could be considered as such, an everyday disease like appendicitis of course could not. Fortunately, Whitehead was not prosecuted for grievous bodily harm or manslaughter, as Price and Smilovitz were able to testify that Houdini had given him permission to punch him.

Among the audience at Houdini's last performance in the Garrick Theater in Detroit on 24 October 1926 was a man called Harry Rickles. He later recalled that the show had been a disappointment. It had started more than half an hour late and Houdini did not look well. He made mistakes, so that the audience could see through his tricks, and he had to be supported by his assistant several times. But when Rickles read that the escape artist had performed with a burst appendix, from which he died several days later, he realised that Houdini had given his life to perform for his admirers right up to the last minute.

10

Narcosis

L'anaesthésie à la reine: Queen Victoria

VICTORIA OF HANOVER was Queen of the United Kingdom and Empress of India. The sun never set on her empire: her children and grandchildren belonged to many of the royal families of Europe and the era in which she reigned was even named after her. She married her cousin Prince Albert of Saxe-Coburg and Gotha and together they seemed like the dream couple, considered the most in-love of all couples in British royal history. Less well known is that they fought constantly, sometimes coming to blows, and it was often the same issue that repeatedly soured the mood in Buckingham Palace. Victoria could not bear the insufferable pain that accompanied what she called the 'animalistic' experience of giving birth. She would become so enraged that Prince Albert finally threatened to leave her if she hit him just once more. Queen Victoria may have been a strong woman, but she felt these assaults on her spirits and her nerves were intolerably sordid. And, although the births of her first seven children had all passed off without problems, she had experienced them as an indescribable trauma. Each was followed by a post-natal depression of at least a year, which ran seamlessly into her next pregnancy. In 1853, Victoria was pregnant again and was again becoming hysterical about the impending drama. Albert decided that this could go on no longer and called in a doctor named John Snow. It was time for anaesthesia.

The technique of putting a patient to sleep, or inducing complete unconsciousness is known as general anaesthesia or narcosis (Greek 'sleep'). The first operation performed under general anaesthesia had, at that time, been performed seven years earlier, on 16 October 1846, at the Massachusetts General Hospital in Boston, United States. A dentist called William Morton had anaesthetised a patient called Edward Abbott, by getting him to inhale ether, diethyl ether to be exact. Abbott had a tumour in his neck that had to be removed. While he was asleep, a surgeon called John Warren cut the tumour out. Everything went well, the patient had felt nothing and simply woke up after the operation. Warren was very impressed, uttering the historic, if understated, words 'Gentlemen, this is no humbug.' It was a turning point in the history of surgery.

Ever since the invention of sharp tools, anyone wishing to help someone else by cutting them open had to contend with the patient thrashing around during the operation. Being cut open is not only painful, but the patient is afraid, above all of not surviving the ordeal. Surgeons therefore always had to be quick, not only to keep the duration of the pain as short as possible, but also because there was little opportunity to take your time while the patient was being held down by your assistants or other helpers. It was therefore a matter of 'the faster, the better'. London surgeon Robert Liston would always start his operations by calling out to his audience: 'Time me, gentlemen, time me!' If you had not completed your work before the patient wrested himself free from the helpers who were pinning him down to the table, the consequences were disastrous. The victim would still be bleeding profusely and, with all the thrashing around and the panic, blood would be spraying in all directions. That would cause the unfortunate patient to become even more terrified and frantic, making it much more difficult to hold him down. This gave rise to a very specific dress code. Until around a hundred and fifty years ago, surgeons would always wear a black coat when operating. That made it less obvious that it was covered in blood and they did not have to wash it so often. Some surgeons used to boast that their coats were so stiff from all the blood that they could stand upright on their own.

So you had to be quick, otherwise it would end badly. Speed meant safety. And that called for short, deep and accurate incisions – in the right place, and passing through as many layers of tissue as possible with one cut. The flow of blood was therefore always stemmed at the end, 'on the way back', by tying off the tissue layers with thread, searing them closed with a branding iron or simply applying a very tight bandage. This method was effective, but not very secure. It left no time to examine closely what you were doing and there was little time or space for unexpected circumstances. So, that was what operations were like until 16 October 1846: quick and bloody – and standardised, with no time for specifics.

Administering a general anaesthetic was therefore considered a waste of time for a quick surgeon and, in Europe, it took a long time for it to become regular surgical practice. Many surgeons were openly opposed to what they saw as dangerous and unnec-essary nonsense. Anaesthesia was known in England as 'Yankee humbug' only good for quacks who were not good enough to operate quickly. But that was to change, thanks to the temper of Queen Victoria. After she had dared to try anaesthesia and had benefited so tremendously from it, no one could dismiss it any longer. It was exactly the boost that this new, unknown, but welcome discovery needed to convince the public at large.

John Snow was a farmer's son and amateur anaesthetist who had written a book about ether and chloroform and designed a special mask to administer chloroform slowly and in controlled doses. In 1847, a year after the first ether anaesthesia was performed in Boston, James Young Simpson performed the first chloroform anaesthesia in Edinburgh. What John Snow did in 1853 was thus nothing new, but it was rare. Did Victoria know that Snow was

Anaesthesiology

Today, anaesthesiology is rightly a full-scale discipline in itself. The days of a few drops of ether on a handkerchief are long over. Three kinds of medicine are used in modern general anaesthesia. A narcotic reduces consciousness, causing sleep (narcosis) and forgetfulness (amnesia). As the narcotic does not completely repress physical reactions to the pain of the operation – such as increased heartbeat and blood pressure, goose bumps and sweating – powerful painkillers (analgesics) are also administered. These are often opium derivatives. Anaesthesia means literally 'without feeling'. To repress the tensing of the muscles in response to manipulation during the operation, a muscle relaxant is often included in the cocktail. These are derived from curare, the poison that Amazonian Indians use for their arrows. This combination of three medicines results in a relaxed, sleeping patient with no physical reactions to the operation. The anaesthetist uses a ventilator, a respiration machine to take over the patient's breathing, inserting a tracheal tube into the windpipe (trachea) via the nose or mouth (intubation). While the patient is under general anaesthetic, the heartbeat, oxygen content in the blood, and carbon dioxide content in the exhaled air, are continually monitored via a blood pressure band and electrodes on the chest and finger. During the operation, the anaesthetist checks a lot more, including the blood count, urine production, blood-sugar level and blood coagulation. The stage of putting the patient to sleep is known as 'induction', and the waking stage as 'emergence'.

not actually an expert, or that he didn't know the risks of what he was going to do to her, or her unborn child? Snow's heart must have been pounding as he climbed the stairs to the royal bedrooms in the palace. It was evening and the corridors, reception rooms and stairways were illuminated by gaslight. The staff would have been nervous. The cabinet was on stand-by, the people waited in suspense and there, beyond the antechambers and yet more doors, Snow would have heard the queen moaning. No doubt, Snow would have wondered whether the queen was able to receive him, a complete stranger, a commoner, calmly and with respect. When he entered, he would have positioned himself at the head of the bed and, not permitted to use the dosing mask he himself had designed, laid a clean handkerchief over Her Majesty's nose and mouth. Using a pipette, he would have dripped a few droplets of chloroform from a bottle onto the handkerchief. He would certainly also have inhaled a little of the chloroform – that is unavoidable – so he would have turned his head to the side now and again to breathe deeply clean air.

Snow recorded every detail. He administered the chloroform to the queen, drop by drop, until she indicated that she felt no more pain, noting that the chloroform had no impact on the contractions, which remained just as severe. From twenty minutes past midnight on 7 April 1853, he gave Victoria fifteen drops of chloroform on the handkerchief with every contraction. 'Her Majesty expressed great relief from the application,' he wrote, 'the pains being trifling during the uterine contractions, and whilst between the periods of contraction there was complete ease.' The queen was not for one moment stupefied by the chloroform, and remained conscious throughout the birth. The child was born 53 minutes later, at 1.13 in the morning. The placenta followed a few minutes later, and the queen was delighted, '. . . expressing herself much gratified with the effect of chloroform'. She herself described it as '. . . that blessed chloroform, soothing and delightful beyond measure'. The newborn prince was christened Leopold; he was their eighth child and fourth son.

Albert was over the moon, though their delight didn't last long: shortly afterwards, the queen fell into her usual post-natal depression, the worst she had ever experienced. The medical journal the *Lancet* published a damning comment and biblical scholars were outraged as the Scriptures state that women must endure pain when giving birth. But the news came as a bombshell to the wider public throughout Europe. In France, the use of chloroform became immensely popular and was given the catchy name '*l'anaesthésie à la reine*'. Patients no longer wished to be operated on without anaesthesia and surgeons were forced to comply with their demands.

Within a few decades, the days of the old, quick surgery were over and a new order emerged. Thanks to anaesthetics, surgeons now had time to work more precisely, and they were no longer distracted by their patients thrashing around and screaming in pain. Operations became precise, meticulous and dry, with no noise, and no blood spattering everywhere. Incisions were careful and exact. Tissue was no longer cut through in one go, but layer for layer, with the flow of blood being stemmed before the following layer was cut open – 'on the way' rather than at the end. And with new heroes like Friedrich Trendelenburg, Theodor Billroth and Richard von Volkmann, surgery became a precision science. Black surgery coats were replaced by white ones.

One of the great new names was the American William Halsted. An innovator in treating inguinal hernias and breast cancer, Halsted had introduced rubber gloves in surgery and with a number of colleagues he had put together a working group to develop local anaesthesia, a wonderful new invention. The procedure, which entailed injecting an anaesthetic drug around a nerve, allowed the patient to remain awake, but to feel nothing in the anaesthetised, numb area. The group met regularly to practise on each other and enjoyed wonderful evenings together. Halsted became not only a pioneer of local anaesthesia, but – because the drug they used was cocaine – he also became an addict. Cocaine has long since been replaced in local anaesthesia by derivative drugs that have the same effect locally, but without the stimulating side effects.

Anaesthesia was a revolution in surgery; the next step was the introduction of hygiene. In 1847, the Hungarian Ignaz Semmelweis discovered that childbed fever – an infection contracted by mothers shortly after childbirth – occurred when medical students returning from the dissecting-room after practising anatomy on dead bodies did not wash their hands before assisting with births. No one believed, however, that something as simple as washing your hands could make the difference between life and death and Semmelweis was dismissed as mad. (It did not help that he unfortunately suffered from a neurological disorder that was gradually driving him insane.) Semmelweis's basic principle of hygiene was not accepted until Louis Pasteur exposed bacteria as the cause of disease and Joseph Lister was the first, in 1865, to prevent the infection of a surgical wound by using an antiseptic. Though revolutionary, these methods were, initially, very painful, because of the corrosive effect of disinfectant in the wound and the length of time they took to administer. They could therefore only be applied thanks to the invention of anaesthesia.

The chloroform that so delighted Queen Victoria was abandoned in the twentieth century, after it was discovered that it could damage the liver and cause irregular heartbeat. Ether, too, was replaced by something else: nitrous oxide (N_2O), also known as laughing gas, a powerful anaesthetic. But it too went out of use when it proved to be a significant greenhouse gas 300 times more damaging to the environment than carbon dioxide.

In modern anaesthesia, the drugs are injected directly into the bloodstream, which means they take effect more quickly and the dose can be more precisely adjusted during the operation. The most commonly used anaesthetic drug at this time is 2,6-Diisopropylphenol, better known as propofol. Propofol has significant advantages and the effects wear off quickly once it is no longer administered. And even better, when patients wake up, they feel as though they have slept very soundly. Because of its milky appearance, it is also known as 'happy milk' or 'milk of amnesia'. But this miracle anaesthetic is not without risks: pop star Michael Jackson became addicted to propofol and died after using it in 2009, because the doctor who administered it to him had not paid sufficient attention to Jackson's state of health. That is a real medical error; as a good anaesthetist will ensure that a patient is closely monitored for twenty-four hours after waking up.

We do not know whether John Snow was able to monitor his patient in this way. And despite his services to the queen, Dr Snow is not remembered as a great anaesthetist. He is, however, remembered for a completely different reason. In 1854, he described an outbreak of cholera in London, identifying a single public water pump as the source of the infection. He was the first to show how a disease can be contagious, and the founding father of epidemiology, the study of how diseases spread.

Victoria insisted that Snow be present, with his anaesthetic, at the birth of her next child on 14 April 1857. It was a girl, Princess Beatrice. And, much to everyone's surprise, this time the queen did not suffer from post-natal depression. Beatrice was her ninth – and last – child.

11

Gangrene

The Battle of Little Bay: Peter Stuyvesant

O N HIS SECOND voyage westward in search of India, the first land that Christopher Columbus saw rising up on the horizon was an island that he named after that day, Dominica (Sunday). He sailed on, to the north-west, and arrived eight days later at another island, which he again called after the day it was sighted, Monday 11 November 1493. But Columbus had of course not discovered new land. People had already been living there for thousands of years. The original inhabitants, the Carib Indians, called their island Soualiga, which means 'salt-land'. From 1627, Dutch ships regularly visited the island for the salt that was extracted from an extensive salt pan between the hills overlooking a large bay. In the seventeenth century there was great demand for salt in the Netherlands to preserve herring. To gather it, there were plenty of slaves available from the adjacent island of Sint-Eustatius, where they arrived directly from Africa to be shipped to further destinations in the New World. The Spanish, however, still considered the island to be theirs. What's more, they were at war with Holland and were not prepared to tolerate the Dutch grabbing 'their' salt. In 1633, they reoccupied the island and built a number of forts. One of these was on the headland that extends far into the sea between Great Bay and the adjacent Little Bay. From there, they made life difficult for the Dutch *fluyts*, the ships carrying the salt. In 1644, the director of the West India Company in Curaçao came to resolve the situation.

Today, the island – incidentally not called Monday but Saint Martin, as the day on which Columbus sighted it (11 November) is St Martin's Day – is loved for its thirty-four excellent beaches. Peter Stuyvesant could therefore have chosen thirty-three other beaches for his attack on the island. But he wanted to conquer Little Bay, as it gave access to the Spanish fort. Stuyvesant knew that if he could take that beach, where tourists now lie in the sun and go snorkelling in the crystal clear turquoise water, he could take the whole island.

Stuyvesant was no great strategist. The attack was an utter disaster for the Dutch troops and a painful humiliation for him personally. His ships had taken many days to sail the 500 nautical miles across the Caribbean Sea from the distant Leeward Islands to Sint Maarten. They encountered no resistance at all when the *Blauwe Haan*, Stuyvesant's flagship, approached the island and, on 20 March 1644, Palm Sunday, entered Cay Bay, a small inlet just past the beautiful Little Bay. They crossed the shallows to the shore in rowing boats. Proudly, the Frisian minister's son stepped into the warm water and strode up the beach. Under the command of Jacob Polak, the governor of Bonaire, the men dragged a cannon up the hill overlooking Little Bay and the Spanish fort on the headland on the other side. But Little Bay was too big, or the cannon was too small, and the cannonballs did not reach the fort. So they had to find an emplacement closer to the target. With a flanking movement, Stuyvesant led the way to a hillock directly above the beach of Little Bay, called Bel-Air. There, he planted the Dutch flag, well within range of the cannons in the Spanish fort immediately in front of him.

Boom! The first shot the Spaniards fired was a direct hit and shattered Stuyvesant's right leg. The captain of the *Blauwe Haan*, who was standing next to Stuyvesant, was also hit and lost a cheek and an eye. Stuyvesant was immediately carried off, rowed back to the ship and hoisted aboard.

What we, fortunately, have not had to face for a very long time must have been immediately clear to Peter Stuyvesant as he lay groaning in the sloop. He may not have dared to look at his leg, but he would immediately have understood – whatever the seriousness of the injury or the size of the wound – that it would have to be amputated. Until about a hundred and fifty years ago, amputation was the only effective treatment for an open leg fracture. Even if the wounds were less complex, the consequences of not amputating immediately would usually be fatal, as gas gangrene – the greatest adversary of wound healing – was always a danger.

The word gangrene is a general term to describe the dying off of living tissue. It is the terrifying final stage of a shortage of oxygen in the skin, the subcutaneous tissue, the muscles or even an entire limb. Although the dead tissues feel as cold as ice, the victim develops a high fever. Gangrene can be caused by a blocked artery. You could then speak of an infarction. That leads to a sharply defined black mummification of part of the limb. The dead part dries out. That is referred to as dry gangrene. But tissue can also die off due to infection of a wound. Because of the pus and the rotting fluids that this produces, it is called wet gangrene. Some bacteria also produce gas, resulting in a form of wet gangrene called gas gangrene.

Gas gangrene is the deadliest form of gangrene and is mostly caused by a micro-organism with the appropriate name *Clostridium perfringens*, from the Latin verb *perfringere*, which means 'crush', 'demolish', 'assault' or 'break through with violence'. It can be found everywhere on the planet. Sand, soil, faeces and street refuse are full of it. *Perfringens* comes from a dangerous family. *Clostridium tetani* causes the lethal disease tetanus, or 'lockjaw', *Clostridium difficile* a life-threatening great bowel infection and *Clostridium botulinum* deadly food poisoning. In unhygienic conditions, *Clostridium perfringens* also causes the much-feared childbed fever, which unnecessarily cost the lives of so many women in childbirth in the past.

The *Clostridium perfringens* bacteria is an anaerobic life-form, meaning that it only survives in an oxygen-free environment. The bacteria has two dangerous properties: it emits rotting gases and produces toxic substances known as toxins. For many centuries, surgery was frustrated by gas gangrene and wound infections. But why does one wound become infected and another not, and why would gas gangrene have developed in Peter Stuyvesant's wound? And why does it hardly occur in the present day?

Three elements determine whether an infection or gangrene develop in a wound. Firstly, of course, there has to be a wound. The size of the opening in the skin is not that important. Bacteria are small enough to enter through even the smallest wounds. The second determining factor is the quantity of bacteria that succeed in multiplying in the wound. That can be minimised by cleaning the wound and keeping it clean. But most important is the damage to the tissues surrounding the wound, called the 'wound bed'. The state of the wound bed is crucial to what follows.

In a wound caused by a sharp knife, the wound bed will hardly be damaged. The edges of the wound will remain unharmed and the healthy tissues will allow the immune system to kill any bacteria that enter the wound. A clean cut with a sharp knife can even be closed up again immediately, if you rinse it out quickly with water, soap or disinfectant. This is primary healing or healing in the first instance (*per primam*). If the cut is not clean, the wound will become infected, producing pus. The infected wound can then no longer be closed up *per primam* and will have to heal *per secundam*, through secondary healing or 'healing in the second instance'. However, the healthy wound bed also guarantees a sufficient supply of oxygen. As the *Clostridium perfringens* bacteria cannot survive in the presence of oxygen, gas gangrene has little chance in a healthy cut, no matter how dirty the wound may be.

In the case of a crush wound, by contrast, the tissues are damaged by bruising, crushing or tearing. Consequently, the blood vessels in the wound bed are also damaged, reducing the supply of oxygen. That will cause much more tissue to die off than the size of the wound would suggest. This dead tissue is referred to as necrosis and provides an ideal breeding ground for all kinds of bacteria. But, because of the lack of oxygen in the wound, the *Clostridium perfringens* bacteria will thrive the most. That is how gas gangrene starts.

For anyone who knows all this, the solution is relatively simple. Clean the wound as quickly as possible. Rinse it out with clean water (for example, the crystal clear sea water in the bays of Saint Martin) and leave it open. Then use a sharp knife to cut away all the dead material until you come to healthy tissue. There are fine-sounding surgical terms for this: *debridement* or *nettoyage* in French, *anfrischen* in German, or *necrosectomy* in English (from the Latin/Greek). Then keep the wound clean until it is fully healed, *per secundam*.

Unfortunately, in the past surgeons always did exactly the opposite. Rather than cleaning wounds by rinsing or washing, they burned them. That does kill the bacteria, but also the tissues and blood vessels in the wound bed, increasing the shortage of oxygen. Surgeons also treated the resulting fever by bloodletting, causing anaemia and thus restricting the supply of oxygen to the wound even more.

Peter Stuyvesant's wound had even more collateral damage. The impact of the cannon ball had shattered his bone, which protruded through the wound. Stuyvesant's leg had undoubtedly become a veritable feast for the minute *Clostridium perfringens*. In these conditions, the anaerobic bacteria would have been able to multiply very rapidly. The immune system responds to such an attack with an inflammatory reaction, causing fever and the production of pus. The microbes then produce toxins that kill the still healthy cells in their vicinity. That generates rotting juices that, together with the pus, form wet gangrene. The rotting gas

Knives and forks

Just as a knife, fork, spoon, glass and serviette are standard attributes at the dining table to enable us to enjoy a meal, standard instruments are required on the operating table to enable a modern operation to be performed. A surgical knife – formerly a one-piece scalpel – now consists of a handle into which disposable blades can be clicked. That means the blade is always sharp, clean and undamaged. Various blades can be used, indicated by a number. The most commonly used are the number 10 (large, curved blade), the number 15 (small, curved blade) and the number 11 (pointed, stabbing blade). Tissue is held with tweezer-like forceps. There are blunt 'anatomical' forceps and atraumatic 'surgical' forceps with pointed ends. There are scissors to cut or spread tissue and scissors to cut thread. The suture needle is held in a special clamp, known as a needle holder. The wound is held open with retractors. The blood is wiped away with sterile gauzes of different sizes. Rinsing fluid and disinfectant are kept in small bowls on the instrument table and there is a wide range of clamps, in all shapes and sizes, for all kinds of uses. For bone operations, there are screwdrivers, saws, gouges, chisels, drills, hammers and files. There are surgical probes, dilators, specula and suction tubes. Stapling machines in wide varieties are used in modern operations to make joins in the abdomen between the stomach and the intestines. Lastly, almost no operation can be performed without electrocoagulation, using an electric probe to cut or sear tissue.

exuded by the bacilli comes under pressure and forces its way into the healthy tissues, which are consequently cut off from their blood supply. The gas can be felt under the skin, and is crunchy, like walking in fresh snow. The gas and toxins kill more and more tissue and the infection spreads more quickly. As the amount of dead tissue increases, the supply of oxygen decreases further, making the environment progressively more favourable for the pathogen. This mass attack was always fatal.

Peter Stuyvesant's wound was full of *Clostridium perfringens*. They were in the soil of Bel-Air, on the cannonball that had lain on the ground on the Spanish side, in the dirty sloop that had taken him back to the ship, on the dirty hands of the surgeon and in the black edges of his fingernails, on the dirty operating table, on the surgeon's dirty saw and in the dirty bandages. The ship's surgeon did not know all that, but he did know that an amputation could save Stuyvesant's life, if he did it high enough up the leg, in the healthy tissue. For him, it was a routine operation, for which he needed four instruments.

The patient was laid on the table. The surgeon applied a tourniquet to the upper leg. That served not only to stem the flow of blood, but also to somewhat numb the leg. After half an hour, it would cause the patient sufficient pins and needles to distract him from the pain of the cut.

The surgeon then took the amputation knife. This was not a small instrument like a scalpel, but a kind of butcher's knife, 30 centimetres long and 3 centimetres wide, razor sharp, with a pointed end and a sturdy handle. He used the knife to cut through to the bone in one go, just above the knee. The cut alone was of course enough to cause excruciating pain, but it was mainly when the surgeon sliced through the large nerves, that run right down the leg like thick cables, producing a sudden, icy pain that would certainly have made the patient scream in agony. Placing a piece of wood between Stuyvesant's teeth to bite on helped to dampen that awful sound.

Between the muscles, tendons and nerves run the major blood vessels, which of course also had to be cut through. Thanks to the tourniquet around the upper leg, the blood did not spurt out, but the bandage could not prevent the blood vessels from emptying out on the other side. The lower leg contained about a litre of blood, which now started to flow out of the amputation wound over the table, so that everything was soon covered in blood.

The cut had to be made in the healthy part of the leg, well above the wound caused by the cannonball. But the bone had to be sawn through a little higher still, so that the end could be well covered with muscle and skin. The next step was therefore to scrape the muscles from the bone, over a length of about a hand's width. The surgeon did that with a scraper with the rather macabre name 'raspatory'. He scraped away the periosteum, the membrane covering the bone, with four or five forceful strokes, as though he were planing a piece of wood. That would have been met with four or five horrendous screams from the patient, if he had not by now lost his voice. Then the surgeon took the saw. With a robust, sharp saw, you can cut through the thigh bone with less than ten strokes. The patient would have felt the vibrations of the saw teeth literally 'to the bone'. Bone dust, blood, vomit, urine and sweat, all mixed together – it would have been a filthy mess. And then there would be a solid thump as the leg fell away. A leg is surprisingly heavy, much heavier than you would expect. Or perhaps surprisingly light if you no longer have it.

The stump was left open and wrapped thoroughly in bandages, after which the tourniquet could be removed. If the wound continued to bleed, the surgeon could always use the branding iron. The patient had long ago fallen into a dead faint anyway. The open wound healed *per secundam*.

Tens of thousands of legs must have been removed in this way in the history of warfare. The record is held by Dominique Jean Larrey, a surgeon in the French army, who is alleged to have performed 700 amputations in four days during the Battle of the Sierra Negra in 1794 in Spain. That amounted to around four minutes for each leg, if he had been sawing all day long for four days. He was able to do this thanks to an invention that still bears his name, the Larrey retractor, a shield that could be opened and fitted around the bone, so that the muscles and the skin could be scraped off with one firm tug, leaving the way clear for the saw. That made the scraping with the raspatory unnecessary. The unfortunate victims were probably lined up and fitted with a tourniquet. Then came Larrey with his knife and retractor, followed by an assistant with the saw, and another with the bandage.

That we no longer have to apply this standard procedure is thanks to a macabre experiment conducted on an unsuspecting eleven-year-old orphan. Little James Greenlees had fallen under a coach in Glasgow. His shinbone was broken and was sticking out through the skin. The wound was full of the dirt from the street. Without amputation, he would certainly have died, as gangrene would have developed. Yet Joseph Lister spared the boy an amputation. On 12 August 1865, rather than cutting off the leg, he sprayed the wound with a corrosive liquid, carbolic acid. This experimental treatment proved successful, James's life and his leg were saved, Lister was made a lord, and antisepsis – the use of antiseptics to treat wounds – was born. No one asked whether the manner of this discovery was justifiable. It was apparently quite normal to experiment on children.

Peter Stuyvesant's defeat was a fiasco. The Spaniards must have laughed out loud. But the Dutch refused to give in and, in the days that followed, made a series of further futile attempts to attack the Spanish fort, from the land and from the sea. One of the ships deployed was the *Blauwe Haan*, on which Stuyvesant was recovering from his amputation. It was hit by three cannon-balls. On 17 April, exactly four weeks after they had arrived, the Dutch retreated with their tails between their legs and the island of San Martin remained Spanish for another four years.

Peter Stuyvesant returned to the Netherlands. With one leg,

he was no longer fit for the life of a seagoing merchant, so the company gave him a desk job on shore. He was made director-general of the colony of New Netherland, where he became the first mayor of New Amsterdam, a settlement on the island of Manhattan. An amputation clearly did not always mean the end of a career. However, a regular seaman who had lost a limb could not usually count on such a favourable return to duty. They would usually be discharged and end up as beggars on land or go back to sea as pirates.

In 1664, the village of New Amsterdam was captured by the English, who would rename it New York. Stuyvesant went back to the Netherlands, but returned to New York later to live as a normal citizen. He died there in 1672, at the age of sixty-one, and is entombed in St Mark's Church in-the-Bowery.

In 1648, the Dutch retrieved Saint Martin under the terms of the Peace of Münster. At least, half of it. The French colonised the north of the island (Saint-Martin) and the Dutch the south (Sint Maarten). But, although both colonies lived in harmony for nearly four centuries, everyone on the island speaks English. The magnificent salt-pan behind Great Bay is now home to the national landfill site.

12

Diagnosis

Doctors and Surgeons: Hercule Poirot and Sherlock Holmes

THERE WERE TIMES that, when visiting patients, doctors did not so much as lift a finger to examine them. Perhaps they felt they were too good for such mundane concerns, or were afraid of catching a disease themselves. Patients in Asia and Arabia used a figurine of wood or ivory to point out where they felt pain. Whether the doctor listened to them is a different matter. Often, even that was pointless, as doctors had no effective treatment to offer. What they prescribed was always the same: enemas via the anus, purging via the mouth and a panacea, a medicine that would help against all complaints, such as the cure-all theriac, a pill made of Venetian snake cookies. The contrast with the surgeon was enormous – he did everything with his hands. And his treatment was much more specific than that of a doctor. After all, there is no panacea in surgery – you can't treat one complaint with an operation for a different one.

Fortunately, much has changed in medicine. Treatment by non-surgical doctors became equally valuable and specific. Yet, a gap has always remained between the two professions regarding involvement with the patient's illness. Non-surgical doctors are expected to make a correct diagnosis, i.e. determine what is wrong with the patient. The best treatments for most diagnoses have now been found. Diseases are treated with medicines according to fixed protocols and guidelines. The doctor then simply has to wait for the patient's own healing powers to do their work. If the patient does not make it – and the diagnosis was correct – there is nothing you can do.

For surgeons, it is different. The success of an operation depends not only on the right diagnosis, a protocol and the patient's own healing powers, but also on the surgeon's personal involvement in the treatment. If the patient doesn't make it and the diagnosis was correct, the surgeon still could have made an error. This means that surgeons, much more than non-surgical doctors, become personally involved in the patient's illness. The surgeon is literally part of how the disease ends, happy or not.

This has led to a situation in which surgeons seek to establish what is wrong with a patient in a different way from non-surgical doctors. Because, as a surgeon, you have to answer to yourself for the fact that a patient's recovery depends on your skill, you want to be absolutely sure what is wrong with him before you start. That need for certainty is far less urgent for non-surgical doctors. They can afford to be more distant from the beginning.

How do you decide what is wrong with a patient? In other words, make a diagnosis? Throughout the history of medicine, doctors have tried to answer that question. From the very beginning, they have always been confronted with the patient's fear. Anyone feeling that their end is nigh, wants to know from the doctor how it will happen. Is there still any hope? How long have I got? Will I suffer pain? To answer these questions sensibly you have to recognise the patient's problem. Doctors could do that better than anyone, because they had seen more diseases and disorders in their lives than other people. Once they knew what a patient had, they could make a prediction. Those two steps were known as diagnosis and prognosis, medical terms derived from the Greek word *gnosis*, meaning knowledge. Diagnosis, with the Greek preposition *dia* (through), means 'seeing through' or 'insight into'. Prognosis, with the preposition *pro* (before), thus means a prediction or a prospect.

It was initially sufficient for a diagnosis to describe a disorder, even if you did not really know what was wrong. And you had no need of your hands to do that. If you saw a few pimples here and there, there was probably not much wrong, no matter what it was. But if the patient was covered from head to toe in badly smelling oozing pustules, that was something to be concerned about. In both cases, you could prescribe simple household remedies. If they didn't help, they also did little harm.

For many centuries, the lack of understanding of the underlying causes of diseases was glossed over with a rather insubstantial story about four alleged bodily fluids, or humours: blood, mucus, yellow bile and black bile. The belief that a disease or complaint arose because the humours were out of balance was not, however, a good starting point for a surgeon. The only way for any of the four fluids to be replenished or reduced in quantity was by bloodletting, and that had very dubious effects. It was a typical remedy of non-surgical doctors.

The next step is not only to recognise and name the problem, but to find out what is causing it. Surgeons want to remove the causes, preferably with a knife. A diagnosis is important for the prognosis, while a cause is important for the treatment. Ileus, for example, is a general term for an obstruction in the passage of food and faeces through the intestines. It is a good example of a diagnosis dating from the time before we had any understanding of causes. If there is nothing you can do about it, the prognosis following a diagnosis of ileus is always bleak, no matter what the cause. The patient begins to vomit, is unable to defecate or break wind, develops a swollen abdomen, complains of severe cramps and, if the symptoms do not pass, will die. But if you can do something about it, you need to know not only that it is indeed ileus, but what has caused it. The intestine may be obstructed by a tumour or an inflammation, but also by a chicken bone. The diagnosis remains the same, but the surgical treatment is different in each case. The question asking what is wrong with a patient therefore embraces a number of other questions: what are the patient's symptoms, what has caused them and how has that led to the disease?

Because a modern diagnosis entails much more than it used to, the search for the answer has become more and more of a challenge, requiring highly developed skills. Medical doctors and surgeons work in the same way as detectives trying to solve a crime. A doctor trying to find out what is wrong with a patient resembles a detective searching for the perpetrator: identifying the cause of a disease is like looking for the motive for a crime, and establishing how a disease could have developed is reminiscent of following the tracks of the murderer and asking how he used the murder weapon. Just as all real detectives have their own style, doctors also solve mysteries in different ways.

The best writer of detective stories was undoubtedly Agatha Christie and by far the most brilliant character in her books was the detective Hercule Poirot. Poirot is an eloquent man, charming and intelligent, who unerringly solves every mystery that comes his way. But his creator also depicts him as something of an anti-hero. He is polite, but also vain and conceited; objective, but also arrogant and moody; inquisitive, but only willing to help if he finds the case interesting enough, and, though he speaks French, he is Belgian. The respectable, middle-aged detective is an eccentric, astute and prosperous man with a smartly waxed handlebar moustache, who time and time again – much to the killer's chagrin, of course – happens to be in the vicinity when a murder takes place. In the Hercule Poirot stories, the plot unfolds according to a fixed formula. Poirot is surrounded by a company of well-defined characters at a more or less self-contained location – a remote country house, the Orient Express stranded somewhere in the snow, or a boat on the Nile. A murder takes place that must have been committed by someone in the group. As Poirot investigates the murder, it is clear that he knows more than he lets on. In the final chapter, he gathers everyone together in the drawing room or the saloon, to reveal the identity of the killer. He then addresses each of them individually. He explains that each one of them could have committed the murder. Each proves to have a hidden motive and no one has a cast-iron alibi. The butler had the key and access to the knife, the baroness had debts and could therefore make good use of the inheritance, the kitchen maid was jealous – nothing is too outrageous.

After having discussed the motives of each character, however, Poirot presents a counter-argument showing that he or she did not commit the murder. Until he comes to the final one – the killer. But that does not become clear until he has first been through all the others individually. In this way, the tension is built up until Poirot comes to the last remaining character and reveals the circumstances surrounding the horrific murder. His detailed accounts of the potential involvement of each character are so fascinating that we easily forget that the majority of the information he has gathered in fact has nothing to do with the case. After all, only the story about the real killer is relevant to solving the mystery.

This is exactly how an internist works. An internist is a non-surgical doctor, a medical specialist in General Internal Medicine (GIM) who concerns himself with diseases and treats them with medicine. A pulmonologist (who specialises in lung diseases), for example, is an internist, as is a gastroenterologist (digestive system), a cardiologist (heart), a nephrologist (kidneys) and an oncologist (cancer). Internists treat diabetes, cardiovascular diseases, blood diseases, inflammatory diseases, in fact all kinds of diseases, as long as an operation is not required. Like Hercule Poirot, an internist prefers to solve problems with a list. Poirot starts his analysis with the crime, asking 'What happened?' An internist starts with the patient's complaint and asks 'What is the problem?' Then they both isolate the problem and restrict themselves to a well-defined summary of potential culprits. Poirot asks himself which of those present could have committed the murder, while an internist asks himself what might be the possible causes of the complaint. This is known in medicine as drawing up a differential diagnosis. Agatha Christie usually made it easy for Poirot to draw up his list by limiting the number of people at the scene of the crime, but internists too no longer have such a difficult time as formerly in drafting a differential diagnosis. Medicine has advanced so far in the past fifty years that, for most complaints and disorders, it is easy to look up a list of possible causes in a manual, in summary articles, in the medical-scientific literature or on the Internet. An internist thus has a list of differential diagnoses ready in no time.

Then it is time to analyse the evidence and clues. Poirot interrogates and investigates and, if necessary, calls others in to assist. An internist also questions his patient, not only about his current complaint, but also his general state of health, his medical history and family. He examines the patient, requests supplementary tests – blood tests, for example, or X-rays – and will, if necessary, ask the advice of a specialist in another area. Essentially, both Poirot and the internist focus on all potential perpetrators, and not only on the most likely ones.

Lastly, they have to exclude the unlikely culprits. They look closely at each of the candidates to see whether he or she could be guilty. They go through the whole list until there is only one left – the least unlikely. For the detective, it is the main suspect, for an internist, it is referred to as a 'working diagnosis'. Exclusion on the basis of probability can lead to very surprising conclusions in the Poirot stories. In *Murder on the Orient Express*, for example, all those present prove to be guilty, while in *Death on the Nile*, the victim himself is the guilty party.

Surgeons do not understand this way of working. Their reasoning is usually more pragmatic and linear. Women may come from Venus and men from Mars, but it sometimes seems to surgeons that internists live in a completely different universe, far removed from all earthly logic. A surgeon can, for example, become very hot under the collar when an internist asks him to 'exclude ileus' in the case of a patient who no longer displays any symptoms and should actually be discharged, just because the radiologist happened to see what 'could be interpreted as a possible ileus' on the CT scan of the patient's abdomen. For an internist, a result like this upsets his checklist and a suspected ileus must therefore be excluded by a surgeon. For a surgeon, however, that is nonsense. It is immediately clear that he should not operate on a patient with no symptoms simply on the grounds of a suspicion.

Conversely, an internist can be equally irritated by a surgeon who, while operating on a patient with suspected acute appendicitis, discovers that the small intestine is inflamed, rather than the appendix. Inflammation of the small intestine is not treated surgically, but with medicine. Yet the surgeon will stand by his decision to operate, because he found the patient very ill and suspected that he was suffering from life-threatening peritonitis. The internist could present arguments in return that throw doubt on the probability of appendicitis. For example, that the patient had been suffering from diarrhoea for a week before the inflammation occurred, which makes the diagnosis less likely.

What lies behind this mutual lack of understanding is a philosophical distinction between deduction and induction, two ways of discovering the truth through logic. Historically, the deductive is older than the inductive method, but both were replaced in the philosophy of science by the scientific method, developed by Karl Popper in 1934.

During the Middle Ages, it was widely believed that human knowledge had already reached its zenith in the golden age of classical antiquity. Doctors and surgeons therefore based their work uncritically on the wisdom of the Greek philosopher Aristotle and the Roman gladiator physician Galen, two men who, with hindsight, did not stand out as providing their theses with a solid foundation in fact. In the Renaissance, scientists once again dared to think critically and drew their own conclusions from general observations. That is deduction. A surgeon knows, as a general observation, that peritonitis can be fatal and that operating to remove the appendix presents a smaller risk. It is then logical, deductively speaking, to conduct an operation in a specific situation in which you suspect the patient may be suffering from appendicitis.

During the Enlightenment, a century later, the experiment developed as a serious basis for science. Conclusions were drawn from specific findings. That is induction. The more indications there are of a certain phenomenon, the more probable it is, and vice versa. A diagnosis of ileus is more probable if a CT scan shows possible indications of the disease, but less probable if the patient displays no symptoms and even less probable if a surgeon sees no reason to operate.

Then Karl Popper introduced the principle of falsifiability and the scientific method. He stated that the truth cannot be discovered. We can only develop a theory of the truth, and then only if we observe one crucial condition: the theory must be formulated in such a way that it can be refuted. This became the basis of all modern medical science. In daily clinical practice, the scientific method works as follows: a clear treatment plan is set in motion for a patient as quickly as possible, based on a working diagnosis. That working diagnosis is based on a falsifiable theory of reality. If the treatment does not have the desired effect, the working diagnosis must be critically reviewed. To reach a working diagnosis, however, induction and deduction remain at the patient's bedside.

Diagnosis

The investigation of a patient's condition consists essentially of three elements. Firstly, the doctor will ask about the patient's medical history, his current complaints (symptoms) and use of medication. This is known as the 'anamnesis', a Greek term meaning 'from memory'. The doctor will also ask about diseases in the patient's family and may ask other people about the patient (hetero-anamnesis). This might be, for example, the parents of a sick child or bystanders in the case of a traffic accident. The anamnesis is followed by a physical examination, during which the doctor feels, smells, looks, listens and measures. Looking is known as inspection, feeling as palpation, tapping as percussion, and listening with a stethoscope as auscultation. A doctor uses his index finger to palpate the rectum; this is known as *palpatio per anum*. He can test the reflexes of the pupils with a light and that of the tendons with a hammer. He can look in the ear with an otoscope and at the retina with a fundoscope. He can test different forms of feeling with a sharp pin or a tuning fork. A doctor's nose is also an important instrument. You can sometimes determine the nature or composition of pus, wound infections or body fluids surprisingly accurately just by smell. Lastly, the doctor can request supplementary tests, such as a blood test, microscopic examination or medical imaging. Imaging can take the form of, for instance, an X-ray photograph, a contrast medium examination or a CT scan. Other examples of imaging include MRI (magnetic resonance imaging) scans, Doppler, ultrasound scans and duplex ultrasonography. Finally, disorders can sometimes be identified using radioactivity, via an isotope scan. This is known as scintigraphy.

If Hercule Poirot is the master of induction, that other great detective in world literature, Sherlock Holmes, is the master of deduction. Holmes solves his cases in a completely different way, just as a surgeon reaches a working diagnosis differently from an internist. Sherlock Holmes is tall and slim, and stern in appearance. He hardly eats, but smokes all the more for it. He solves mysteries in foggy London, wraithlike and shrouded in secrecy. The basis of his success is the enormous repository of random knowledge in his head. He has studied the meanings of sailors' tattoos, knows the colour and composition of the soil in every part of England by heart, and knows what font is used by each newspaper. These are the general facts on which his deduction is based. The strength of Sherlock Holmes's method is observation. 'The world is full of obvious things which nobody by any chance ever observes,' he says, courtesy of his spiritual father and creator Arthur Conan Doyle – who was also a doctor. He uses deduction to compare what he observes with what he knows. He leaps from observation to observation, moving forward all the time. And, because he does it so well, he rarely has to look at other possibilities or change tack. His method is therefore much more efficient than that of Poirot, more direct, but also more vulnerable as success depends on how well he observes and how much he knows. That is why he works alone. He does have a companion, his friend Dr Watson, but Holmes treats him more as a kind of pupil, from whom he expects little assistance. Watson seems to have been conjured up by Conan Doyle purely to allow the thoughts in the detective's lonely mind to be translated into a dialogue, so that the reader can also benefit from them.

It is immediately clear that deduction relies entirely on what is in the mind of the detective or the surgeon. By comparison, induction is much more complex, but is also more transparent and objective. Sherlock Holmes could afford not to go into detail about many of his deductions and only explain the whole thing at the end, because his adventures almost always ended in success. Medical specialists, including surgeons, can no longer permit themselves such a luxury. The times when Sherlock Holmes, superior and unfathomable, could outsmart a criminal in the London fog are now over. A modern surgeon no longer presents himself as an individually focused expert who determines the quality of the investigation into a patient's problem all on his own. Difficult decisions are increasingly made in multidisciplinary consultation, where specialists from various disciplines discuss patients on a case-by-case basis and decisions are thoroughly justified and recorded. The days of deduction are therefore numbered and, who knows, perhaps surgeons and internists will begin to understand each other in the not too distant future?

But one thing will never change. Once a surgeon is standing at the operating table, scalpel at the ready, he is completely alone and everything that he does from that moment, everything that happens to his patient, remains his own, personal responsibility. Then you want to be sure of what you are doing, and you do not help your conscience by working on the basis of probabilities.

13

Complications

The Maestro and the Shah: Mohammed Reza Pahlavi

URING THE SECOND World War, German actress and singer Marlène Dietrich warmed the heart of many a soldier in the front line with her sensual song *Ich bin von Kopf bis Fuß auf Liebe eingestellt*' ('I am, from head to toe, ready for love'*). That was quite a statement from a woman with such long legs. It was even claimed that she had the most beautiful legs in the world. In photographs, she was often portrayed with a cigarette in her hand and that famous sultry expression on her face. All those cigarettes eventually led to the arteries in those beautiful legs clogging up and Dietrich had to be operated on by a vascular surgeon. In her eyes, there was only one man good enough to be permitted to work his magic on her world-famous pins: Michael DeBakey.

A vascular surgeon is a surgeon who specialises in blood vessels, and arteries in particular. Vascular surgical techniques of joining together arteries and veins were devised and tried out in the early years of the twentieth century by just one man, French surgeon Alexis Carrel. Carrel's contribution was considered so important to the advance of general surgery that he was awarded the Nobel Prize for Medicine in 1912. The conditions under which vascular operations are carried out are exceptional. As blood vessels are relatively small, the needles and thread used in

---

* The English title is 'Falling in Love Again (Can't Help It)'

operations must be smaller than those used for other parts of the body. And because blood spurts out immediately if you cut open a blood vessel, it has to be temporarily clamped shut. But the clamps must not stay on for too long, as a limb or organ cannot go without blood for very long. Moreover, once blood stops flowing it can coagulate. And, even after the blood vessel has been sewn up and the blood is flowing again, it can be clogged up again by blood clots on the stitching in the wall of the vessel. Because healthy blood vessels are essential for the survival of organs and other body parts, there is often a greater sense of urgency surrounding vascular operations and a successful operation often feels more like a rescue. No wonder, therefore, that it was a vascular surgeon who was considered an international hero by so many celebrities in the twentieth century.

Vascular surgery was new and exciting and opened up the way to the ultimate organ, the heart. The development of cardiac surgery, operations on the heart, led to a feeling of omnipotence in the surgical world and when the ultimate peak was reached in 1967 – the first successful heart transplant by Christiaan Barnard in Cape Town – it was of the same order as the first moon landing two years later. Michael DeBakey, cardiovascular (heart and blood vessels) surgeon at the Methodist Hospital in Houston, had been at the centre of all these developments. He had conducted groundbreaking work and was involved in the development of the first artificial heart. But he was especially a pioneer in the treatment of a less common disorder, aortic dissection – a very complex problem for a vascular surgeon. Aortic dissection occurs when a tear develops in the inner layer of the aorta, the main artery in the body, which originates in the heart. The blood is forced at high pressure through the tear and between the inner and outer layers of the aorta, which are pushed further and further apart. This is not only very painful, but also threatens the supply of blood to the brain, the arms, ultimately, the rest of the body. DeBakey's operation made it possible to cure this dramatic problem.

DeBakey was known as the maestro. He acquired worldwide renown (and his nickname) thanks to his most famous patient, former King Edward VIII of Great Britain, who went to America unannounced in 1964 to be operated on by DeBakey. Like Dietrich, Edward was a heavy smoker – as indeed most of a vascular surgeon's patients are. At this point Edward was seventy years of age and needed what at that time was a life-threatening vascular operation. But he did not go into any detail with the media, saying only 'I came to see the maestro.' When Russian president Boris Yeltsin needed a quintuple bypass operation thirty-two years later, in 1996, he clearly did not entirely trust his Russian cardiac surgeons and had the now eighty-seven-year-old maestro flown over from America to assist them. Boris called DeBakey 'the magician'. All of the other celebrities who were DeBakey's patients – King Leopold III of Belgium, King Hussein of Jordan, Hollywood stars Danny Kaye and Jerry Lewis, multi-millionaire Aristotle Onassis, American presidents Kennedy, Johnson and Nixon, and Yugoslav dictator Tito – must have shared this opinion. It also did no harm to Michael DeBakey's reputation that he was anything but modest and enjoyed his fame.

So when Mohammed Reza Pahlavi, the deposed Shah of Iran, had to undergo a splenectomy (surgical removal of the spleen) in 1980, in his eyes there was only one surgeon on the planet who could do it. The fact that, as a cardiovascular surgeon, DeBakey actually had nothing to do with the spleen, was apparently not relevant, either for himself or for his esteemed patient.

When the shah fled the revolution in Iran on 16 January 1979 and boarded a plane in Tehran never to see his home country again, he was not only threatened with death by Ayatollah Khomeini and the Islamic rebels but also by cancer. His exile was to become not only a wandering quest from one country to another, where he was always unwelcome, but also a fight against malignant non-Hodgkin lymphoma in his abdomen.

The shah was treated by the French oncologist Professor Georges Flandrin, who followed him from one country to another. An oncologist is an medical specialist in general internal medicine – not a surgeon – who specialises in treating cancer. Flandrin's patient suffered continually from anaemia and pain and, to make things worse, had developed an infection of the gall bladder. He underwent a cholecystectomy, surgical removal of the gall bladder, in New York. The American surgeons confirmed that the shah's liver, and more especially his spleen, were enlarged as a consequence of his malignant disease. He had a hepatosplenomegaly, a medical term that literally means simultaneous enlargement of the liver and the spleen. The large spleen meant that his blood cells were continually broken down; it was also the cause of his pain. The shah recovered reasonably well from his gall-bladder operation, though his admission to the hospital led to demonstrations and riots outside the building, and he and his family no longer felt safe in America. The problem with his gallstones had been solved, but that had no impact on his illness. His pain and fatigue increased and the time came to remove his enormous spleen.

Shortly afterwards, there was a hostage drama in the American embassy in Tehran and President Jimmy Carter probably wanted to be rid of his high-ranking guest as quickly as possible. The shah and his wife, Empress Farah Diba, moved on to Mexico, the Bahamas and Panama, but everywhere they went, the threat of extradition hung over their heads. An operation could not be carried out under these circumstances. But President Sadat of Egypt was willing to offer his old friend shelter and medical care, so in March 1980 the shah arrived at the Maadi Military Hospital in Cairo. Five days later, DeBakey arrived with his assistants, an anaesthetist and a pathologist. On 28 March, the operation to remove the spleen was performed by two surgeons, DeBakey and the Egyptian Fouad Nour. The patient's wife and eldest son watched the operation live via a television connection with the operating room. The operation went well and, according to DeBakey, the shah's spleen was as large as an American football.

The spleen has relatively little function in the body and you can afford to lose it, if necessary. It plays a role in maintaining the quality of the blood by filtering out old blood cells and, especially at a younger age, is part of the body's immune system. Because you can sometimes feel a strange sensation near the spleen when running or when you get the giggles, Pliny the Elder thought that the function of the spleen had something to do with these activities. There are two references to splenectomies performed in the sixteenth century. In 1549, Adriano Zacarelli is recorded as having removed a young woman's spleen in Naples and, in 1590 Franciscus Rosetti allegedly removed half a one, again in Italy. It seems unlikely, however, that these operations really did remove the spleen, as the first abdominal operation in which the patient survived was not carried out until 1809. More probably, in both cases, it was a large clot of blood resulting from a deep subcutaneous contusion. Such a clot can closely resemble the spleen, with the same colour and the same solid texture, explaining why the two Italians thought the clots they had removed were spleens. The first genuine successful splenectomy was performed in Paris in 1876 by Jules-Émile Péan. It was the spleen of a twenty-year-old woman and weighed more than a kilogram.

A splenectomy does not have to be a difficult operation, as long as you stick to the rules. The procedure can be learned in the third or fourth year of training to be a surgeon. There are a couple of things to watch out for, but the spleen itself is relatively straightforward. It is normally the size of half an avocado and looks a little like a toadstool, with the blood vessels carrying blood to and from the organ on one side, resembling the toadstool's stalk. But it is difficult to get at, hidden away deep in the top left of the abdominal cavity. You have to stick both hands into the abdomen past your wrists to reach it. And the spleen is very delicate. If you pull or push it too hard, it can rip, which is dangerous as a spleen can bleed heavily. And if it ruptures, you can easily lose sight of it because of all the blood, so you have to avoid that at all costs. And then there is the final warning that surgeons give when teaching the operation: watch out for the tail of the pancreas!

The pancreas is an elongated organ, described in German as the 'abdominal saliva gland'. The digestive juices that the pancreas produces, however, are much more aggressive than saliva. They digest, for example, the meat in our food. The tail of this organ runs alongside the blood vessels of the spleen and can extend as far as the spleen stalk. If you place the clamp on the blood vessels of the spleen a little too far to the right, you not only remove the spleen, but also a piece of the pancreas. That can be very dangerous, as pancreatic juices can leak into the abdominal cavity and literally digest the tissues of the body, producing pus. With a normal spleen, it is fortunately not overly difficult to place the clamp correctly and spare the pancreas. But the shah's splenectomy was especially difficult because the organ was so big.

Nour had asked DeBakey, 'Isn't the tail of the pancreas caught in the clamp?' But DeBakey dismissed his Egyptian colleague's observation with a wave of the hand and tied the tissue under his clamp with a large ligature. Nour cautiously suggested at least leaving a drain behind, a small tube to allow any excess fluid to run out of the abdomen, just in case, but DeBakey thought that was unnecessary and closed the abdomen without a drain. He was applauded when he removed his gloves. The spleen weighed 1,900 grams. Cancer was found in the spleen and in the pieces of liver that had been removed for testing. Unfortunately, the microscopic study also found pancreatic tissue . . .

The third day after the operation, the patient developed pain in the back of his left shoulder and a fever. But the wound from the operation healed quickly and the shah was able to walk in the garden of the hospital again when DeBakey left for Houston. There, he allowed himself to be interviewed like a hero, but his patient, far away, was slowly deteriorating. The fever refused to go away and the shah felt sick and tired. He had little pain, but lay in bed the whole day.

The fever continued unabated for several months, day after day. The shah was given blood transfusions and antibiotics, a procession of American doctors came and went, but DeBakey himself remained in Houston and had X-ray photographs sent over. He guessed that the shah had pneumonia in the lower left lung. A bronchoscopy was performed – an unpleasant examination of the airways – but no problems were found. The many specialists involved had completely lost sight of the big picture and, in Paris, Professor Flandrin followed the situation with mounting amazement. Did no one see that the patient simply had an abscess under his diaphragm?

It is a classic cause of error in surgery: an infection in the abdominal cavity produces fever and irritation of the peritoneum, unless the infection is located below the diaphragm. Then the only symptom is fever. The medical term for 'under the diaphragm' is subphrenic. Pus under the diaphragm is therefore referred to as a subphrenic abscess. If a patient has an infection in the abdominal cavity and the peritoneum is irritated, he will experience severe pain, which will increase with the slightest movement; this is an overtly clear indication for every doctor. But if only the diaphragm is irritated and not the peritoneum, these telltale symptoms do not arise. The patient suffers only a fever, with perhaps the hiccups, or pain in the shoulder. Flandrin saw this, and he was not even a surgeon. Even the X-rays of the lungs fitted the picture. He decided to do something about it, flew to Egypt and started arguing with everybody. He had a surgeon,

Pierre-Louis Fagniez, flown out from France. On 2 July, Fagniez made a small incision in the upper left of the shah's abdomen and drained a litre and a half of pus from the abdominal cavity. The shah had thus been left for three months with a large abscess below his diaphragm. He immediately felt better, was able to walk around, got his appetite back and started to concern himself with affairs of state again. But three and a half weeks later, he suddenly collapsed. His blood pressure fell, he became deathly pale, and he lost consciousness. He was given blood, but not operated on. The shah died unexpectedly of internal haemorrhaging on 27 July 1980. He was sixty years old.

He had been suffering from Waldenström's macroglobulinaemia, a rare, not very aggressive form of non-Hodgkin cancer that can develop in the liver and the spleen. Yet this was not the cause of the shah's death; that was due to the damage to his pancreas during DeBakey's splenectomy. That complication was iatrogenic, i.e. 'caused by a doctor'. The leakage of pancreatic juices after the surgeon had snipped through the tail of the pancreas had led to infection of the large hollow cavity below the diaphragm left behind after removal of the large spleen, which had filled with pus. The aggressive pancreatic fluids would then have eaten away at the wall of the splenic artery, which could lead to sudden arterial haemorrhaging in the upper abdomen.

This account clearly shows how complications after an operation can be life-threatening, but not necessarily fatal. Most complications can be treated successfully, if they are recognised in time and the correct action is taken. They only become life-threatening if they continue for too long or if one complication leads to another. In the case of the shah, both of these things happened. The pancreas was damaged, leading to the development of an abscess. That was treated far too late, haemorrhaging occurred and the unfortunate patient died.

Fever

Human beings, all other mammals, and birds are warm-blooded. Our bodies continually burn energy to keep our temperature at around 37°C. Our thermostat is buried deep in the brain, in the hypothalamus. It can be disrupted by a protein called interleukine-6, which is released by an inflammation. That causes fever, by raising the setting of the thermostat. The body then has to work harder to keep warm and feels too cold. The hypothalamus passes this incorrect information on to the brain, so that we feel cold, even though that is not the case. We start to shiver and shake, while the thermostat raises our body temperature. When, after a time, the impact of the interleukine-6 reduces, the process is reversed: the temperature falls, we feel too warm and start to sweat. It is not clear whether fever performs a function. Should we let it run its course and do its work, though we do not know what that is, or should we fight it and try to cool the patient down? Fever always has a cause, but it can sometimes be difficult to find. Different inflammations have different patterns of rising and falling temperature. A virus infection typically generates a high fever of over 39°C, and a bacterial infection between 38 and 39°C. If bacteria cause an abscess containing pus under pressure, short peaks of high fever also occur, especially in the evenings. Fever resulting from pus will only disappear if the pus is removed surgically. Tuberculosis produces little fever but it does cause profuse sweating, especially at night. A typhoid infection creates a pattern of fever peaks known appropriately as 'brontosaurus fever'. A bladder infection produces no fever at all.

Michael DeBakey lived to be very old. When he felt a pain in his chest on 31 December 2006, at the age of ninety-seven, he almost reconciled himself with the fact that he would die of a heart attack. But when he noticed that the pain persisted and he was still alive, the father of aortic dissection surgery realised that he himself had an aortic dissection. He became the oldest patient to undergo the complex major operation that he himself had developed. And he survived the ordeal. Two years later, just shy of his century, he died a peaceful death.

Special forceps that he designed, the DeBakey forceps, are still used by surgeons around the world on a daily basis. DeBakey was genuinely a great surgeon and an example for many of his colleagues everywhere. But clearly, even great surgeons can sometimes make a mistake. Complications are, after all, part and parcel of operations and the risk of problems can never be counted out, no matter how great you are.

Marlène Dietrich also lived to a great age. She died in Paris in 1992 at the age of ninety – thanks to DeBakey – with two healthy legs.

14

Dissemination

Two Musicians and Their Big Toes: Lully and Bob Marley

CONDUCTORS DID NOT start using the small baton that is so familiar today until the nineteenth century. Before that, they would stand in front of the orchestra beating time with a long staff, topped with a ludicrous, decorative ball. The maces waved around by drum majors at the front of marching bands hark back to that practice. Jean-Baptiste Lully, court composer to the French King Louis XIV in Versailles, also used a long staff when conducting. On Saturday 4 January 1687, while banging his staff on the floor in time to the beat, he suffered an unpleasant industrial accident which, seventy-seven days later, was to cost him his life.

The baroque age was at its peak. Versailles was the centre of the world and, in that centre, Lully was the master of baroque music and French opera. His boss, the Sun King, had just survived an operation on his anus, two months previously. Lully was to perform his *Te Deum* at the beginning of the new year to celebrate the king's recovery. Especially for the occasion he had reworked the sacred ode, originally composed in 1677, into a magisterial master-piece. It was to be performed for the king and a large audience on Wednesday 8 January in the Église des Pères Feuillants in Paris. The Saturday before was the final rehearsal. Trumpets and cymbals echoed through the empty church. There were fifty musicians and a choir of more than a hundred of the best voices in the country. In front of them stood Lully, his long staff taller than himself.

A typical feature of baroque music is the basso continuo, a rhythmic succession of chords providing a basis for the whole piece. The musicians had a certain freedom to improvise, but Lully would have intervened as much as possible in the performance of his own work, and most certainly at rehearsals. With a little imagination, you can see him standing there, passionately keeping the beat of the basso continuo with his enormous staff and demanding the attention of the musicians every now and again by striking the ground. At one such moment, he struck his own toe. Whether Jean-Baptiste clenched his teeth and carried on or screamed out in pain, or whether the musicians and the choir, caught up in the imposing music, noticed nothing of the incident or burst into laughter, we do not know. Perhaps the final rehearsal of the *Te Deum* was interrupted to carry him from the stage, screaming in agony. In any case, the performance of 8 January went ahead, with Lully leading the proceedings, and was a great success. Afterwards, he was seen limping towards his coach and, in the days that followed, his big toe became infected. He developed a fever and his wife sent for a physician, Monsieur Alliot, who advised him to have the toe amputated to prevent gangrene. Lully refused.

The infection spread slowly from the toe to the foot, and from the foot to the leg. Amputation could still have saved his life, and Lully must have known that. And yet, he ignored the wise advice of Dr Alliot and allowed himself to be treated by a quack for the princely sum of 70,000 francs. At first, he recovered, but the fever returned. By then, the charlatan had made off with the money.

Why did Lully refuse the amputation that would have saved his life? Was he too vain to live without a leg? Lully not only wrote operas and ballet, but was also a musician, actor, dancer and choreographer. He was a top entertainer, and not only on the stage. Jean-Baptiste was an Italian of very humble origins, who had worked his way up in France from a simple guitarist to a celebrity. He was a respected composer, husband and father, and a personal friend of the Sun King. But he was also a much-loved character on the Parisian gay scene, who brightened up seventeenth-century France not only with his art, but also with a series of minor and not-so-minor scandals. With only one leg, his career, his pleasure and his status would all have been wiped away.

Or was Lully simply reckless and underestimated the severity of the situation? Seventy-seven days is quite a long time for an infection to ultimately prove fatal. It could not therefore have been gas gangrene, at least not at first, as that spreads like wildfire and, without amputation, will kill you within three days. So it must have been a simpler infection, caused by less aggressive bacteria that spread slowly and with fewer symptoms – perhaps so few that Lully did not see the danger.

The description suggests that the cause was an abscess with lymphangitis and blood poisoning, or a progressive infection that begins as local (the toe), becomes regional (the leg) and then systemic (the whole body). This process of spreading is known as dissemination. An abscess is in essence a closed infection containing pus. What pus is and how it arises has been explained earlier. It is the soup of dead tissue, dead white blood cells and bacteria, which flows from an infected open wound as a creamy, beige-coloured, stinking fluid. But pus can also develop deeper in the body, below the skin. It can then not find a way out and comes under pressure. That causes an abscess. Mostly, with open wounds and closed abscesses, the bacteria in the pus are strep-tococci or staphylococci, which live on our own skin. In the case of an abscess, they must have somehow penetrated into the deeper tissues below the skin. That can only occur through a wound, which is known as the point of entry. It could be a nail that you have stepped on, or a dog bite, an inflamed sebaceous or sweat gland, an ingrown hair, a wound caused by scratching an itch or eczema, or a crack in the skin. With fingers and toes, damage to the cuticle can provide a point of entry, which was probably the case with Lully's toe.

Moreover, Jean-Baptiste's socks would have been swarming with streptococci and staphylococci. Washing or changing your clothes daily was not done in the seventeenth century, and the French court was no exception. There was a good reason why wigs, perfume and toilet waters were so popular. They were necessary to disguise the unwashed hair and the stench of the body and clothing. It was not until a hundred years later, in the time of Napoleon, that some understanding of hygiene developed, leading to the laying of sewers and the provision of facilities for people to wash themselves and their clothes, practices that had disappeared from Europe with the Romans. It is difficult to imagine how filthy the otherwise so colourful life at the court of the Sun King must have been. Jean-Baptiste Lully's sweaty sock must have undoubtedly offered an ideal breeding ground for bacteria.

When an abscess develops, the bacteria below the skin initially only cause an inflammation. The skin swells up and becomes warm, tense, red and painful. But then the bacteria defeat the inflammatory cells and pus forms in the inflammation. At that point, the infection is maturing. The increasing quantity of pus pushes the surrounding tissue away, and the body attempts to halt that process by forming connective or scar tissue. The pus then becomes sealed in by an abscess wall, which temporarily stops the development of the infection. But, because blood can no longer flow to the pus, the immune system cannot combat it. Antibiotics would also have no effect. The patient develops a severe fever and the accumulation of pus feels like a hard ball. If you place two fingers on the swelling and one finger is pushed outwards when you push the other inwards, you know for certain that it is filled with liquid. This is known in surgery as fluctuation. If the swelling fluctuates, the infection is mature and ready to be cut open.

If you cut open the abscess wall and allow all the pus to flow out, the wall has a chance to heal *per secundam* like a normal open wound. This is called incision and drainage. If you do not drain the abscess in time, the bacteria will ultimately break through the abscess wall and be released into the surrounding tissue. That causes an infection of the subcutaneous fatty tissue, known as cellulitis.

The subcutaneous tissues are criss-crossed by minuscule vessels that do not carry blood but tissue fluid known as lymph. These are the lymph vessels, the smallest of which are known as lymph capillaries. In these vessels, lymphangitis develops, an infection that follows the course of the lymph vessels and can be seen on the surface of the skin as a red line leading away from the abscess. This line will be longer each day.

Lymph vessels come together in the lymph nodes, small glands less than half a centimetre across that are found bunched together and act as hubs in the network of lymph vessels. The closest group of nodes to the toe is in the hollow of the knee. The next one is in the groin. The infection causes the lymph nodes to swell up, so that they can easily be felt from the outside as small hard lumps below the skin, the first day behind the knee and the following day in the groin. From the groin, the lymph nodes continue upwards behind the abdomen and finally enter the blood circulation in the chest.

Without antibiotics, an infection of the lymph vessels, lymphangitis, will therefore irrevocably lead to blood poisoning, as large quantities of bacteria will end up in the blood. That will enable them to infect other organs and form abscesses in, for example, the brain, the liver or the adrenal gland. And the whole process will then start again in these abscesses. Whether the patient survives all that will very much depend on his general state of health. A healthy individual will have a healthy immune system and will survive for longer. Lully must have been a healthy man to have held out for seventy-seven days.

Barrier

An important condition for any living thing to survive is being able to maintain a barrier between itself and its environment. That requires energy, which in the case of animal life needs a continual supply of oxygen. A living cell can survive only while its cell membrane is intact. Complex multicellular animals like humans also have barriers to protect them against the outside world, such as skin on the outside, mucous membranes on the inside and the immune system in between. Cancer can develop only if dysfunctioning cancer cells break these barriers down. A good example of barriers being maintained in our body is the pancreas, which can digest meat but − thanks to its own barrier − does not digest itself. The gastric mucosa, the mucous membrane layer of the stomach, even produces pure hydrochloric acid, but is itself resistant to it. Infectious diseases occur when living pathogens break through barriers. That can be caused by an open wound in the skin or mucous membrane, or by an inadequate supply of blood. The latter causes a shortage of oxygen in the body's tissues, which can no longer generate sufficient energy to maintain their barriers. Physical damage and a shortage of oxygen are the main mechanisms leading to barriers being compromised. Understanding these mechanisms is the basis of solving the challenge facing modern surgery − to restore the barrier breached by the scalpel as effectively as possible when performing an operation. This means that the tissues in the area around the operation wound must retain a sufficient supply of blood and, while the wound is open, it must be kept free of living pathogens.

Lully's leg finally turned green and black. He sent first for a notary to draw up his will and then for a priest to hear his confession. On his death bed, this father of ten children, who had been promiscuous with many men, composed a piece of music entitled 'Il faut mourir, pécheur, il faut mourir' (It is time to die, sinner, it is time to die). Lully died on 22 March 1687.

Three centuries later, another great musician died from a disease of his big toe. This man's music was even more influential than that of Lully. He was the father of a completely new musical genre, even though his oeuvre amounts to only a few hours of music. He, too, refused to have his toe amputated, even though it would have saved his life. But, in his case, it was not pride or vanity that held him back. It was that it was not permitted by his religion. And, like Lully, he sought salvation from a quack, who was equally unable to save his life.

It started with a pain in his toe. He could not remember having stubbed it anywhere. At first, he could make the pain bearable by smoking marijuana. For a while, he thought he had damaged his toe playing football, but the pain did not go away. Doctors diagnosed a tumour below the toenail. A small operation was performed to remove the small growth and study it under a microscope. It turned out to be a malignant melanoma, an aggressive form of skin cancer that develops in the melanocytes, the pigment cells in the skin. He was advised to have the toe amputated, but he rejected the advice and decided to tackle the disease by fasting, smoking and using herbal salves. For two years, he ignored the severity of his illness, even when he developed complaints in other places. The cancer in his toe had spread throughout his body. Eventually his symptoms became so bad that he could no longer ignore the fact that he was going to die. He expressed his acceptance of his fate with one of his most beautiful compositions, 'Redemption Song'.

Bob Marley spent the final eight months of his life in Germany, in the clinic of a charlatan who believed he could cure the cancer, which had now spread to his lungs and brain, with a special diet and 'holistic' injections. When the end was near, he wanted to return home to die. During the flight from Germany to his homeland, his health deteriorated further. In Florida, he was too ill to transfer to the plane to Jamaica. He died in a hospital in Miami on 11 May 1981, three years after the diagnosis. The religion that forbade him from defiling his body with an amputation was Rastafari, an important feature of which is to avoid all association with death. Lethal diseases, for example, are therefore denied. Marley was thirty-six years old.

When the body is invaded by cancer, tumour cells spread in the same way as bacteria during an infection. In both cases, a local attack becomes regional and, ultimately, affects the whole body. The mechanism of dissemination is the same. In the case of cancer, this process is known as metastasis, which literally means 'displacement'. Cancer has three malignant properties. The tumour cells escape the body's control mechanisms by moving away from their original position. They are able to find their way through other, healthy body cells. This is known as invasion. How far the invasion of tumour cells has developed is a measure of the stage that the disease has reached. The life cycle of the tumour cells also evades the body's control mechanisms. They multiply indiscriminately, meaning that there are steadily more and more of them. Thirdly, tumour cells lose the properties of the cells they originate from. The less recognisable they are, the more malignantly they behave.

Although tumour cells disseminate through the body in the same way as bacterial infections, they do so much more slowly. Lully survived for seventy-seven days, Marley for three years. Both diseases start locally, where the intruders succeed in penetrating the body's barriers. Bacteria have to wait for their chance and enter the body through damaged skin or mucous membrane, while tumour cells actively force their way through the barriers, even if they are still intact. In both cases – with an infection or cancer – the body is attacked, and takes the form of rapid multiplication of the bacteria or tumour cells and there is active damage to the body's tissues, which provokes a response from the body. The immune system tries to repel the attack. White blood cells, antibodies and macrophages – cells that clean up damage to tissues – combat the bacteria and the cancer cells. At this stage, the attack is still local, extending no further than the place where the infection or tumour originated. The invasion can be stopped surgically by means of total (*in toto*) excision, or resection, of the source. An infected wound with dead tissue (necrosis) can be cut out (necrosectomy), an abscess can be cut open (incision and drainage), and a tumour can be cut away (tumourectomy).

Like bacteria, tumour cells can also disseminate via the lymph vessels to the lymph nodes. In rare cases of tumours in the skin, the spread of cancer through the lymph vessels can be seen with the naked eye, like the red line on the skin visible in the case of lymphangitis. With a little imagination, it looks like a crab: the tumour is the body and the dissemination via the lymph vessels the legs. That is where we get the name 'cancer', from the Latin word for a crab. Mostly, however, the dissemination of cancer cannot be seen with the naked eye.

Tumour cells that spread via the lymph vessels are captured by the lymph nodes, which work like filters. In the lymph nodes, the tumour cells grow to become tumours. The invasion is then no longer local, but regional. At this stage, the enlarged lymph nodes can be felt. As with Lully, this would first have been noticeable with Bob Marley in the hollow of the knee and then the groin. Total excision of the original tumour is no longer effective. A regional excision becomes necessary – in other words, removal of the tumour together with the affected lymph nodes. This is known surgically as a radical excision. The medical term 'radical' comes from the Latin *radix* (root) and means removing something 'by the roots'. As you do not know in advance whether there are already tumour cells in the lymph nodes, you can best remove them all. Surgical resection of cancer must therefore be both total (leaving nothing of the tumour behind) and radical (leaving none of the lymph nodes related to the tumour). Antibiotics can mostly reduce an infection from regional to local level. With some forms of cancer, chemotherapy and radiation treatment can do the same.

Once the intruders invade the circulation system, they can spread to other organs. That is known as 'distant metastasis'. At this stage usually the disease can no longer be treated surgically. Only antibiotics (for infections) and chemotherapy (for cancer) can be effective.

The stages of cancer are classified at local, regional and systemic level, on the basis of the TNM staging system. T stands for tumour. T1 is the earliest stage of the tumour, T3 is a tumour that is growing through the barrier of the organ, T4 means it is penetrating the barrier of an adjacent organ. In most cases, a total surgical resection is possible. The surgeon must then apply a safe margin, removing a few centimetres of tissue around the tumour. This is because the invasion of tumour cells is often more advanced at microscopic than at macroscopic level. N stands for node. No means that the lymph nodes have not been affected by the tumour cells and N1 indicates that the cells have spread to the closest group of nodes. Up to this stage, a radical surgical resection can still cure the disease permanently. N2 usually means that lymph nodes have been affected that can no longer be removed surgically. M stands for metastasis. M0 means there has been no distant metastasis, while M1 indicates that distant organs have been affected. In some cases, such as limited dissemination to the liver, lungs or brain, stage M1 cancer can also still be treated surgically.

The TNM stage of the cancer not only determines the prognosis – how long the patient has left to live – but also the options for treatment. Treating cancer can serve multiple purposes. Curative treatment aims to rid the patient of the cancer completely and permanently. It can then be worth considering the risk of serious side effects or mutilating resections. That is usually only possible in the early stages. Palliative treatment aims to prolong the life of the patient by restricting the progress of the disease or the increase in the number of tumour cells in body. In that case, the benefits – in terms of extra years of life – must be weighed up against the disadvantages of the treatment. The final stage of treatment, end-of-life care, aims to bring the patient's life to an end as comfortably as possible, while doing nothing more to combat the disease.

Based on the advice given to Bob Marley to have 'only' one toe amputated, his cancer must at that time still have been local. Because the small tumour was under his nail, it must have quickly caused him pain, explaining why he discovered the disease in its earliest stage. Surgical resection of a malignant melanoma at this stage (T1NoMo) offers a 90 per cent chance that the patient will still be alive five years later. But Bob Marley refused to give up his toe and did not live to be old. But he did become a legend.

15

Abdomen

The Romans and Abdominoplasty: Lucius Apronius Caesianus

OF ALL POSSIBLE lifestyles, our own Western way of life is most likely to cause obesity. Obesity lies at the root of a wide range of diseases in the modern age, spreading around the world like an epidemic. There is a strong link between obesity and type 2 diabetes, cardiovascular diseases and cancer. The Western lifestyle is therefore an important driver of the steadily rising costs of medical care. And that lifestyle has its origins in ancient Rome. Then too, as now, obesity was a growing problem and, as now, especially among young people. It is perhaps significant that the Romans invented the hamburger.

At the start of the first century AD, Rome was flooded with luxuries from all corners of the empire, at least for those who could afford them. And the most decadent aspect of the lifestyle of the city's wealthy citizens was their eating habits. A slave with a bucket and a feather to tickle the backs of the throats of the guests reclining at table, to arouse a retching reflex to make room for the next course, was a familiar sight at Roman banquets. Roast neck of giraffe, stuffed elephant's trunk, baked hog's womb, dolphin meatballs, fresh deer's brain and peacock tongue pies were actual dishes from the period.

The young Lucius Apronius Caesianus must have enjoyed all these culinary delights. He was severely overweight. His father, Apronius Senior, was a tough, seasoned barbarian-slayer, who had no qualms about punishing a cohort that had shown cowardice in battle by decimation (executing 1 in 10). The region that Julius Caesar had conquered for the *Imperium Romanum* many years before had to be defended, day in day out, against the rebellious peoples in the north. Life in Germania was in stark contrast to life in the city. It consisted of building forts, and attacking and securing positions, and all on a simple, meagre diet of what could be found or caught in the local area: acorns, rabbits, wild boar . . . For this work, Apronius was rewarded in 15 AD with the highest honour granted in the Roman Empire – a triumphal procession in Rome. His career took off, he was a consul for some months and later proconsul of Africa, and the spear with which he had struck a barbarian full in the face was dedicated to the gods. As far as he was concerned, his fat dumpling of a son was seriously in need of a lifestyle change. He was to become a soldier, like his father.

There is only indirect evidence of this conflict between father and son. The great Roman encyclopaedist Pliny the Elder referred to the operation that Lucius had to undergo in his life's work, *Naturalis Historia*, published in 78 AD. In chapter 15 of the eleventh book, on fatty tissue, he writes: 'It is on record that the son of the consular Lucius Apronius had his fat removed by an operation and relieved his body of unmanageable weight.' Pliny mentioned this operation to support his claim that fatty tissue has 'no sensation' and contains no blood vessels. He also wisely notes that overweight animals (and he does not exclude people from this category) do not live to be a great age.

The operation was certainly performed more than once in the Roman Empire, as there is a report from a distant province, in Judea, of a local official in the service of the Romans undergoing the procedure some hundred years after Pliny. According to the account, in the Talmud (Baba Mezi'a, chapter 83b), the patient was the exceptionally corpulent Rabbi Eleazar ben Simeon: 'They gave him a sleeping potion and took him into a marble room and ripped open his abdomen and were taking out baskets of fat . . .' The reason for this operation was not cosmetic but functional. According to the Talmud, Eleazar's belly was reduced in size so that his judgements would be based less on gut feeling and more on good sense. The fat allegedly also obstructed his freedom of movement during copulation.

It is inconceivable that these operations were genuine laparotomies, which involve cutting through the abdominal wall to access the abdominal cavity. Many centuries previously, Hippocrates had written that cutting open the abdomen was always fatal, and the Romans also knew that. In 46 BC, Roman senator Cato had even chosen to cut his abdomen open as a sure way of committing suicide. After a lengthy conflict, Caesar had him cornered in Africa and he decided to end his life. He was found in his bedchamber, still alive. A doctor closed the wound, probably against his better judgement, but during the night Cato picked out the stitches and was dead by sunrise. It would be more than 1,800 years before abdominal operations could be performed successfully.

In times of war, of course, surgeons had to deal with plenty of ripped open abdomens with the intestines spilling out, but the chances of these unfortunate victims surviving were so slight that no self-respecting surgeon would ever contemplate inflicting similar wounds on a patient in peacetime. So what is so dangerous about an open abdomen that it was taboo for surgeons for such a long time? Actually nothing at all. Opening and closing an abdomen is no different from treating any other wound. The danger lay in the complexity found behind the abdominal wall.

Simple folk tales show that early ideas of what happens in our abdomens were not very sophisticated. In reality, you cannot walk into the belly of a whale and then walk back out again a few days later. Nor can you easily free a grandmother in her nightdress, a little girl in red hooded cape, or six baby goats from the

The first laparotomy

The first successful abdominal operation (laparotomy) was performed, remarkably, several decades before the invention of anaesthesia and the understanding of asepsis. Ephraim McDowell, a rural surgeon in America, removed an enormous tumour from the left ovary of a forty-four-year-old woman, Jane Todd Crawford, on Christmas Day 1809, by performing a laparotomy in the living room of his house in Danville, Kentucky. The woman kept herself calm by singing psalms. The operation lasted half an hour and the patient recovered well. She lived a long and healthy life, dying at the age of seventy-eight. McDowell kept a cool head when he opened the abdomen and the intestines spilled out onto the table. He wrote that he was unable to push them back during the operation but, after he had removed the enormous tumour, there was apparently enough room for them again. Today, a laparotomy is the standard procedure for all organs in the abdominal cavity. The abdomen can be opened in various ways: vertically along the centre line, horizontally, diagonally, with a hockey stick incision, a chevron incision, a McBurney's incision, a Kocher's incision, a Battle's incision or a Pfannenstiel incision. A laparotomy can be performed for an infection in the abdomen, a perforation of the gastrointestinal tract, to remove a tumour, or to repair an ileus, an obstruction in the passage of food and faeces through the intestines. The procedure is, however, increasingly being replaced by a laparoscopy, keyhole surgery in the abdomen.

belly of a wolf, fill the belly with stones, and then sew the belly back up again. Apart from anything else, what we eat doesn't end up in the abdominal cavity, but in the intestines.

The gastrointestinal tract is in essence one long tube that runs from the mouth to the anus. The different components of the tube have various functions, structures and names, but it remains one single tube. After the oral cavity (the mouth) comes the pharynx, then the oesophagus, the stomach, the duodenum, the small intestine, the large intestine (colon), which incorporates the caecum and the appendix, and finally the rectum. From the stomach to the rectum, the tube – which is about nine metres long in total – lies folded up in the abdominal cavity. For its whole length, it is connected to the back of the abdominal cavity by an attachment called the mesentery. The stomach and intestines are therefore not completely free within the abdominal cavity. Blood vessels run to the intestines and the stomach through this mesentery. There are four other organs in the abdominal cavity: the liver, the gall bladder, the spleen and the omentum, a large fold of fatty tissue. In the case of women, there is the womb and two ovaries as well. That's it. There is a small quantity of fluid between the intestines and the organs, but no air. The abdominal cavity has not a single connection to any of the body's natural orifices and that is why there are no bacteria in it.

Because the abdominal cavity is almost completely filled with intestines and organs, the bowels lie directly against the abdominal wall. You have to cut the wall open very carefully so as not to damage them. But that has almost always been impossible, for various reasons. The pressure in the abdomen is high because the abdominal muscles are continually under tension. There are four muscles on each side: the *rectus abdominis* (the right and left one together are more popularly known as the 'abs'), which each run vertically, the outer and the inner oblique muscles, which run diagonally downwards and upwards respectively, and the transverse muscle, which runs horizontally. We use all of these muscles to stand or sit upright, and to bend. But the abdominal muscles also tense when the abdominal wall is cut open, as a reflex response to the pain, panic and struggles of the patient. The abdominal wall then presses against the intestines, making it difficult to avoid them with the scalpel. The pressure also makes them spill out through the wound as soon as the incision is made so that, before you know it, they are lying on the outside of the belly or on the table. That, of course, makes life very difficult for the surgeon. The reverse process is just as tricky, because it is almost impossible to push back the intestines of a conscious patient, let alone close the wound up neatly.

In the third century BC, two physicians in Ptolemaic Alexandria called Erasistratus and Herophilus were given permission to investigate the anatomy of the human abdomen by experimenting on living prisoners who had been sentenced to death. They would certainly have encountered the high pressure in the living abdomen, but there would of course be no need to stitch it back together again. What their unfortunate victims underwent must have been horrific, but it perhaps spared them an even more terrible death by torture. They will have noticed that the pain of the incision was followed by pain in the peritoneum, the inner lining of the abdominal cavity that stretches around the intestines and abdominal organs (the word peritoneum means 'stretched around'). It contains nerve fibres, and touching it causes severe nausea and retching. How can you operate effectively while your patient is screaming with pain and starts to vomit every time you touch the inside of his open abdomen? And, if you damaged the intestines when opening the abdomen, their contents and all the bacteria they contain will have spilled out into the abdominal cavity and the patient will die within a few days of peritonitis. So you need a calm patient, who does not feel anything, does not tense up his abdominal muscles and does not start to vomit. And, of course, a surgeon who works hygienically and does not harm the intestines.

In the story from the Talmud, the special marble room in which Rabbi Eleazar was operated on may suggest some idea of the basic hygienic conditions required for surgery. But the operation would certainly not have been performed in the kind of clean environment that is essential for abdominal surgery. The sleeping potion given to the rabbi before the operation is also a hint of some sort of anaesthetic, but it would certainly not have been powerful enough to sufficiently relax his abdominal muscles and anaesthetise the peritoneum. Neither Apronius nor Eleazar could have undergone a genuine operation in the abdomen as both men are known to have survived their operations for many years. In the case of a fat belly, the superfluous fat does not all have to be inside the abdominal cavity – it can also have accumulated subcutaneously, between the skin and the abdominal muscles. If the two men did not undergo operations to remove fat from inside their abdomens, then they must both have had fat removed from around their bellies. In other words, an operation outside the abdominal wall and not in the abdominal cavity. In medical terms, such an operation is known as an abdominoplasty (from *abdomen* and the Greek *-lastos*, meaning moulded or formed). In popular terms, it is called a 'tummy tuck'.

Yet, even that must have been a perilous undertaking in those days. We know now that problems with the wound occur so often if you remove skin and subcutaneous fatty tissue from patients suffering from obesity that abdominal wall corrections are only performed on people who have first lost a considerable amount of weight. In that respect, Pliny was almost correct when he used the operation on Lucius Apronius to illustrate the properties of fatty tissue. Although subcutaneous fatty tissue does contain blood vessels, there are very few of them. That means that the thicker a subcutaneous layer of fat is, the greater the risk of a wound becoming infected or not healing properly.

In Roman times, wound infections were still life-threatening complications. As we know from other sources that Lucius lived a long and healthy life after the operation, the abdominal wall correction clearly proceeded without serious complications in his case. Perhaps he first lost some weight before undergoing the surgical procedure and that what Pliny referred to relieving 'his body of unmanageable weight' did not refer directly to his obesity, but to the layers of excess skin remaining after he had lost weight. We know that Rabbi Eleazar, on the other hand, suffered terrible pain in the final years of his life. Could that have been as a result of complications arising from his operation?

Today, an upper weight limit of 100 kilograms is often applied for those undergoing an abdominoplasty. Howard Kelly, a gynaecologist in Baltimore, described the first abdominoplasty in modern times in 1899. In the 1960s the Brazilian plastic surgeon Ivo Pitanguy, who became renowned for his work on Elizabeth Taylor, developed the cosmetic abdominoplasty. This procedure became the basis of all present variants of abdominal wall correction. In 1982, French surgeon Yves-Gerard Illouz presented a new trick for removing subcutaneous fat using a steel tube and a powerful vacuum. This method, liposuction, involves making a small incision in the skin and pulling the steel tube forcefully back and forth through the fatty tissue, breaking it into smaller fragments and sucking it away. Here, too, Pliny was almost right. Fatty tissue is not completely without 'sensation', but contains so few nerve fibres that liposuction can be conducted under local anaesthesia. The options for corrections to remove excess skin have now expanded enormously, the pinnacle being the 'contour operation', a 360-degree correction procedure. The patient first lies on his or her back and undergoes an operation on the skin of the abdomen and is then turned over while under general anaesthesia onto his 'new' stomach so that the surgeon can also correct the back.

How did life fare for the two heroes of this story? Lucius Apronius did become a soldier and fought alongside his father in Africa. There, far away from the decadence of the city, he apparently had no difficulty in maintaining his healthy new lifestyle. He also reached the highest rank and, in 39 AD, became a consul, together with the Emperor Caligula.

Around two thousand years later the Western lifestyle that had caused him such suffering resurfaced. At the start of the new millennium, one in eight adults worldwide suffer from obesity, and only 5 per cent of those who try to follow in the footsteps of Apronius Junior and radically change their lifestyle succeed in doing so permanently.

Pliny the Elder died during the eruption of Mount Vesuvius in 79 AD, which covered the city of Pompeii with lava. He had tied a cushion on his head for protection against the pumice falling from the sky, but it was to no avail. He suffocated in the smoke. Incidentally he was overweight, at least, if we are to believe his nephew, Pliny the Younger, who recorded the circumstances of his uncle's death.

In this chapter it is assumed that Pliny meant that it was the son of Consul Apronius Senior who underwent the operation. As the son bore the same name, however, and was also a consul before Pliny wrote his anecdote about the operation, it is possible that it refers to an unknown son of Apronius Junior. That would, of course, have made the story much less fascinating . . .

16

Aneurysm

The Relativity of Surgery: Albert Einstein

MODERN SURGERY IS not absolute. It is a science of probabilities and calculating chances. It is probable, for example, that an inflammation of the gall bladder will be accompanied by fever, but it is far less likely that someone with a fever is suffering from an inflamed gall bladder. After all, in general, fever occurs more often than gall-bladder inflammations. The probability increases if another symptom or sign occurs alongside the fever that is typical of an inflamed gall bladder. A third typical symptom or sign will of course make the diagnosis even more probable. A combination of three symptoms or signs is known as a triad. The triad for an inflamed gall bladder, cholecystitis, is fever, pain in the upper abdomen that radiates out to the back, and 'Murphy's sign', tenderness in the right upper abdomen that increases with inhalation. Triads are 'specific', in other words the diagnosis is probable and there is a good chance, if all three indications are present, that the patient is suffering from that illness. But they are mostly not 'sensitive', meaning that the illness can also often occur without the complete triad being present.

Supplementary tests – like a blood test, X-ray or ultrasound scan – have their own sensitivity and specificity, which must be taken into account when interpreting the results. Even a decision to perform an operation (the indication of the operation), is relative and based only on probabilities. The chances of the operation being successful must be weighed up against the risk of doing nothing. These chances and risks are expressed in terms like '30 days mortality' (the probability that the patient will die in the first month after the operation), 'morbidity' (the probability of side effects and complications arising from the operation), the 'recurrence rate' (the probability that the illness recurs) or 'five-year survival rate' (the probability that the patient will still be alive after five years). These degrees of probability and risk are now known for most tests, diseases and operations. Taking account of these percentages is known as evidence-based surgery. In practice, this means that surgical decisions have to be made on the basis of figures published in the medical research literature. That literature can be consulted on the Internet, for example on the website www.pubmed.com, where – with well-chosen keywords – you can find everything ever published in medical journals about a certain medical problem. In modern surgery, therefore, it is not about a clear yes or no, but a greater or lesser degree of probability, with a greater or lesser chance of success.

Of course there are exceptions. Patients who prove that the improbable can occur, by displaying a surprising diagnosis or by surviving against all expectations, are incontestable proof of the relativity of surgery. Albert Einstein, the father of relativity, was one such patient. He had a life-threatening disease of the aorta, but his symptoms resembled those of an inflammation of the gall bladder and he lived longer with the disease than was actually considered possible.

The aorta is the largest blood vessel in our bodies. It runs vertically downwards through the thoracic (chest) cavity and the section of it that passes through the abdomen, the abdominal aorta, is normally some two centimetres in diameter. If the rigidity of the wall of the aorta is compromised, the pressure of the blood flowing through it will cause it to slowly blow up like a balloon. Unlike other cardiovascular disease, there is not always a clearly demonstrable cause. Such an inflation of an artery is called an aneurysm and, in the abdominal aorta, an abdominal aortic aneurysm, or AAA for short. Because an aneurysm does not restrict the flow of blood, it does not usually display any symptoms. And yet, an AAA will eventually rupture and so, once it reaches a certain size, it will need treatment. The AAA becomes an AAAA, an acute abdominal aortic aneurysm, which unlike an AAA, does show symptoms. The sudden strain on the artery, the small tears that this produces in the artery wall and the subsequent leaking of blood cause severe pain, in the abdomen or the back, which without urgent treatment can rupture fully within hours or days. Albert Einstein had an AAA and he had symptoms, but not for hours or days. He had them for many years.

Einstein was twenty-six when he presented his theory of relativity in 1905. It turned the world on its head, and $E=mc2$ became the most famous formula of all time. But fascist ideas and open anti-Semitism were brewing in Europe and by 1933, the year in which the National Socialist German Workers' Party – the Nazis – came to power in Germany, Einstein – who was Jewish – left Germany for America after receiving an attractive offer to work in Princeton, New Jersey. In the same year, Berlin surgeon Rudolf Nissen also fled Germany for Istanbul.

Nissen might not be as well known as Einstein, but among surgeons he is remembered for an operation known as a Nissen fundoplication. This elegant surgical procedure is used to treat gastroesophageal reflux disease (acid reflux), where the contents of the stomach can enter the oesophagus, causing unpleasant symptoms like heartburn and belching. But Nissen had a much greater impact as a general surgeon. In 1931, he performed the first successful resection of a whole lung; he developed the frozen section procedure – a method of performing rapid microscopic analysis of a specimen during an operation – and he was the first to perform a complete resection of the oesophagus. When the

Second World War broke out, he also emigrated to America but, because his qualifications were not valid there, he had to work first as a surgical assistant before opening his own private practice in Manhattan in 1941. A short time later, he accepted a position as chief surgeon in two hospitals in New York, the Brooklyn Jewish Hospital and the Maimonides Hospital, where he built up a great reputation.

It was there, in 1948, that he met his most famous patient. Albert Einstein was then already sixty-nine years old and had never had health problems, though he smoked a pipe his whole life, never played sport and had gained some weight in recent years probably due to his famously unhealthy eating habits. Einstein consulted Nissen because, several times a year, he had pain in the upper right of his abdomen, which lasted for a few days and was mostly accompanied by vomiting. These were symptoms that could easily be caused by gallstones. The triad for a gallbladder attack is pain in the upper right abdomen, nausea or vomiting and an inability to sit still. But Einstein explained how this time he had also fainted in the bathroom of his house in Princeton – a symptom that was no longer typical of gallstones. An X-ray showed no signs of stones in the gall bladder and during the physical examination, Nissen felt a pulsating mass in the centre of the abdomen. He feared that it might be an aneurysm of the abdominal aorta and that what Einstein had experienced in his bathroom – sudden pain and fainting – could be symptomatic of an AAAA. In that case, the patient was risking imminent death if he were not operated on.

Today, this is a standard operation with good results and an acceptable risk, certainly in the case of a relatively young patient of sixty-nine. Its success, however, depends on two preconditions that could not be fulfilled in 1948. Firstly, before the operation X-ray studies have to be made to determine the size (diameter), the extension (length) and the location of the aneurysm (in relation to the arteries of the kidneys). Today, that takes the form of a CT scan with a contrast medium and an ultrasound scan, but, in 1948, these methods had not yet been developed. Nissen therefore had to plan the procedure during the operation itself. Secondly, he actually had little treatment to offer his patient. The first successful operation to replace an AAA was not performed until 1951 in Paris, in which surgeon Charles Dubost used a piece of aorta from a deceased donor. In the event of an acute ruptured aneurysm in 1948, a surgeon could tie off the aorta to save the patient's life, but, as that cuts off the supply of blood to the legs they would die off. In Albert Einstein's case, such a horrendous complication was unthinkable, as his life did not seem to be in danger.

When Nissen performed the abdominal operation on Einstein, he found a normal gall bladder with no stones, but also an aneurysm of the abdominal aorta the size of a grapefruit. As the aneurysm was still intact, Nissen applied an experimental method: he wrapped it in cellophane. The idea was that the cellophane – the same synthetic material used to wrap sweets, bread and cigars – which was alien to the body but completely soluble, would stimulate a connective tissue reaction, resulting in the formation of scar tissue that would strengthen the thin wall of the distended artery and perhaps postpone the inevitable rupture for some time.

Cellophane, a transparent cellulose polymer developed in 1900, has a wide variety of uses and experiments were carried out to explore its potential in surgery. Although the method had already been used for some time, the long-term results were not yet clear. And it required guts to wrap the aneurysm of the greatest scientist of all time in what was essentially a sandwich bag. In the years following Einstein's operation, the use of cellophane was completely superseded by vascular prosthetic surgery, in which the diseased section of the aorta is replaced by a plastic tube.

Today many a vascular surgeon will laugh heartily at the mention of cellophane in surgery. And yet, Albert Einstein lived for another seven years with his neatly packaged grapefruit aneurysm. With what we now know about AAAs that is a small miracle.

Nissen probably did not estimate the size of Einstein's AAA randomly. Doctors frequently used fruit to describe the size of a 'space-occupying lesion' like a tumour or an aneurysm. The mandarin, orange and grapefruit were especially popular because they indicated a diameter of two, three and four inches, respectively. Nissen would have chosen his fruit carefully, as the larger the aneurysm, the worse the prospects for the patient. An average grapefruit is ten centimetres in diameter. The median survival of patients with an untreated AAA larger than seven centimetres is only nine months, which means that half of these patients die before that. The annual risk of an aneurysm larger than eight centimetres rupturing is more than 30 per cent, year in, year out. With an aneurysm of ten centimetres, therefore, Einstein should have been dead within one or two years. His chances of surviving for seven years were only a few per cent.

Despite the perilous situation that Einstein was in, he recovered quickly from the operation and left the hospital just three weeks later. Four years after his operation, he was even offered the presidency of the state of Israel. In the final seven years of his life, Einstein, whose scientific research had not produced any more great breakthroughs since his theory of relativity, was still at work at the Institute of Advanced Study in Princeton. But while he tried in vain to reconcile the laws of gravity with those of quantum mechanics, the physical Law of Laplace – a law that says the tension on the wall of an aneurysm, at a constant pressure, is proportional to the diameter – was at work on his aneurysm. The larger the aneurysm, the more tension the same pressure exerts on the wall, and so an aneurysm not only tends to get bigger, but also to get bigger more quickly as the wall of the aneurysm becomes progressively thinner and the risk of a rupture rises.

Stitches and knots

Surgeons can tie knots in a thread very quickly and neatly, with one finger, with both hands, or using a needle holder. There is a special surgeon's knot, a variant on a reef knot, where you begin by turning one thread twice around the other, rather than just once. You then pull the thread tight, holding the knot flat. The double twist will help stop the knot from coming loose, while you tie a single knot on top. When you pull the whole knot together, the double thread will crumple up, pulling the first part of the knot even tighter. All the twists will prevent it from slipping. The most commonly used knots in surgery, however, are simple jamming knots. By not pulling the knots tight, but tying them one after the other on the same thread, the whole knot can still be slipped, allowing the tension to be adjusted knot for knot. The final knot is then pulled tight in the other direction, 'locking' the whole knot. The simplest stitch is a single loop: you pass the needle and thread from the outside to the inside and, on the other side, from the inside to the outside, and finish off with a knot. To approximate both edges of the skin as precisely as possible, surgeons use the 'Donati stitch'. After making a simple stitch, the thread is not yet tightened. The needle and thread are passed back through the skin, but now only one millimetre from the edges on both sides. And then you finish off with a knot.

In April 1955, Einstein experienced abdominal pain again, this time with fever and vomiting. He was seventy-six years old. Although everything once again pointed to an inflammation of the gall bladder (the full triad was present), doctors were naturally afraid that it was an AAAA. By 1955, it was possible to treat an aneurysm with a vascular prosthesis and Frank Glenn, a vascular surgeon from New York who had experience with this procedure, was asked to come and discuss the operation with Einstein. He visited the professor at home and suggested the operation, but Einstein declined the offer. 'It is tasteless to prolong life artificially,' he said, 'I have done my share, it is time to go. I will do it elegantly.' Einstein was given morphine and admitted to Princeton Hospital. Two days later, during the night of 17 April, he died. His exceptional clinical symptoms of a rupturing aneurysm with the triad of an acute inflammation of the gall bladder were named the 'Einstein Sign', in his honour.

So did Nissen's trick with the cellophane work after all? Probably not: Einstein was just lucky. The following day, pathologist Thomas Harvey performed an autopsy on the body of the world-famous scientist. He observed smoker's lung, hardening of the arteries, an enlarged liver and a ruptured abdominal aorta aneurysm, with at least two litres of blood in the abdomen. The gall bladder was normal, but the professor's brain weighed 1,230 grams, 200 grams less than the average adult male.

17

Laparoscopy

Endoscopy and the Minimal Invasive Revolution

FTER A SCIENTIFIC meeting at the Josephinum, the medical academy in Vienna on 9 December 1806, seven gentlemen withdrew to a small back room, where an assistant had laid out the body of a young woman. The professors were to use the corpse to test a device developed by a German doctor, Philipp Bozzini from Frankfurt.

Bozzini called the device – comprising a candle, a speculum (a medical instrument used to inspect bodily orifices) and an ocular lens (the eyepiece that you look through on a microscope or telescope) – a 'light conductor'. It promised to be a remarkable invention. Every doctor knew that the design of the speculum was flawed. Ideally the speculum, the light source and the eye were all aligned to prevent shadows, but then either the candle was in the doctor's way, or the doctor's head obstructed the light – and the candle caused the device to be too hot. But when the Herr Direktor, the Herr Vizedirektor, four honourable professors and the Herr Stabsarzt (staff physician) used Bozzini's device to inspect the vagina and anus of the body on the table they noted delightedly: 'The light conductor sent from Frankfurt by Dr Bozzini was presented and inspected, and it was decided to test it directly on a female corpse that had been laid out for this purpose. The results were promising beyond expectations.'

Although Hippocrates and the surgeons of the ancient world already used specula to examine bodily orifices, this satisfactory experiment with the 'Frankfurt light conductor' is now seen as the real birth of endoscopy, a technique that allows doctors to look inside the body with sufficient light. In the years that followed, the light conductor was improved by doctors and instrument-makers in various countries. In 1855, French surgeon Antonin Jean Desormeaux called his improved version an endoscope, which gave the name to the discipline: endoscopy, 'looking inside'.

Almost 190 years later, on 9 February 1996, after his annual symposium on laparoscopic surgery in the Sint-Lucas Hospital in Assebroek, a suburb of Bruges, Belgian surgeon Luc Van der Heijden is sitting a little nervously at a small table at the front of the auditorium. For this official occasion, he has changed out of his operating clothes and put on a smart suit. Television cameras are focused on him and technicians are trying to make contact with the Sint-Antonius Hospital in Nieuwegein, 150 kilometres away in the Netherlands. The communication link has been made possible by relatively new technology, the Integrated Services Digital Network (ISDN). Dutch surgeon Peter Go appears on the screen. The image is a little shaky and the sound is tinny as he explains that his patient is already anaesthetised and ready on the operating table. He has a groin hernia, which is going to be repaired by laparoscopic (keyhole) surgery. The camera in the patient's abdomen will not be held by human hands, however, but by a robot – and Van der Heijden is going to operate it from Belgium. While the members of Go's operation team in the Netherlands stand with their arms folded in front of them, with the press of a button in Belgium the camera moves up and down and from left to right in the man's abdomen.

Although the laparoscopic hernia repair was eventually completed by the Dutch surgeon Go, this remote operation of the camera was the world's first experiment with telesurgery. Now, twenty years later, complex operations – such as removal of the rectum, the adrenal glands, parts of the large intestine, or a gastric bypass

– are performed laparoscopically as standard procedure. That means they can be performed more quickly (usually within one or two hours) more safely and more easily than was the case with a conventional, open operation. How did we get to this stage?

You don't get far with an instrument that requires lighting a candle, and in 1879 Viennese instrument-maker Josef Leiter and urologist Maximilian Nitze solved the problem once and for all by moving the light source from outside the body, to inside the bodily cavity itself. Leiter and Nitze developed a cystoscope, an instrument that enabled them to look inside the bladder through the urethra with the use of a glowing wire (this was almost six months before Thomas Alva Edison would invent the light bulb) to produce light, which was cooled with water. The cystoscope made Leiter world famous. He persuaded the assistant of the greatest surgeon in the world, Theodor Billroth in Vienna, to help him develop the ultimate endoscope: a gastroscope, an instrument to look inside the stomach. Leiter and the assistant, Johan von Mikulicz, constructed a tube with a water-cooled light on the end. As the patient had to swallow the long tube in its entirety, von Mikulicz performed the first gastroscopy on a circus sword-swallower in 1880. Von Mikulicz would use the gastroscope to examine the stomachs of hundreds of patients, sometimes together with his pupil Georg Kelling.

An examination with Von Mikulicz's rigid tube must have been a terrible experience for the patient. He would be laid on the table on his back, with his head hanging over the edge. Then the metal tube, which was a good 60 centimetres long, would be pushed through his open mouth, down his oesophagus and into his stomach. The stomach was then made visible by pumping it up with air and switching on the light. If the patient lay still, did not panic or choke, the doctor would have enough time to inspect part of the stomach. Not much, but more than anyone had ever dreamed of until then.

Towers and trocars

A laparoscopic operation relies entirely on technology. It requires four devices, which are mostly stacked on top of each other on a movable trolley known as a laparoscopy tower. At the top is the screen, and below the camera unit, to which the handheld digital camera head is connected, is the insufflator, which inflates the abdomen to a constant pressure with carbon dioxide, and the light source. Three cables run from the tower to the operation: the cable from the camera, a fibre-optic cable for the light, and a tube for the carbon dioxide gas. The camera and the light cable are connected to the laparoscope, a tubular instrument about 10 millimetres in diameter and 30–40 centimetres long, with a lens system for the image and light. To gain access to the inflated abdominal cavity, devices called trocars are inserted through the abdominal wall. These are tubes between 5 and 12 millimetres in diameter with an airtight valve, through which the laparoscope, clamps and other instruments can be placed in the abdomen. Electricity is used for cutting and cauterising in the abdomen. That is why the gas in the abdomen may not contain any oxygen and all the instruments and trocars are electrically insulated. The trocars and the laparoscopic instruments are minute and mechanically complex, and as they are easily damaged and difficult to clean, many are disposable and are discarded after each laparoscopy. That makes laparoscopic surgery expensive, but that is paid back by the fact that patients spend less time in hospital.

The next milestone was actually a by-product of a different idea. Experiments inflating the abdominal cavity with air had been carried out for many years in a process known as insufflation; it was tried as a treatment for tuberculosis in a time when experimentation was all that could be done to combat wasting diseases, and it was even alleged to have been successful in some cases.

Either way, it had become clear that inflating the abdomen with air could do little harm. Von Mikulicz, too, had experimented with insufflation and had used the same air pump for his gastroscope. His assistant Georg Kelling had come up with the idea of raising the air pressure in the abdominal cavity higher to stop internal haemorrhaging in the abdomen, and had experimented with this treatment on dogs.

First, Kelling generated a rupture of the liver in the test animal. Then he inflated the abdominal cavity and waited. But the dogs kept dying. He did not understand why the idea would not work and wanted to know exactly what happened in the abdominal cavity. So he inserted a Nitze-Leiter cystoscope through the wall of the inflated abdomen to see it with his own eyes. What it showed was that the air pressure did not press the rupture in the liver closed at all. As he watched the dog bleed to death, he realised he had invented something new.

On 23 September 1901, Kelling repeated the experiment in front of an audience at the 73rd Congress of the Naturalist Scientist's Medical Conference in Hamburg, but now without rupturing the liver. He inflated the abdominal cavity of a healthy dog with air, inserted a cystoscope through the abdominal wall and keyhole surgery was born.

It is difficult to imagine that laparoscopy, which is now irrevocably part of modern surgery, was once completely the domain of non-surgical internists. When Kelling performed that first laparoscopy experiment in 1901, there were few options for supplementary tests to support a diagnosis. Blood tests were still at an embryonic stage, X-rays did not show much of value when it came to the abdomen, and microscopic study was only possible after a patient had died. Laparoscopy was therefore a welcome new method that facilitated significant progress in medicine but which, as yet, had little to do with surgery, and was instead used to examine the liver and other organs close up to determine how far a disease had spread. And the procedure was not without teething problems: in 1923, an abdomen inflated with oxygen briefly caught fire, fortunately doing little damage to the patient. Since then, carbon dioxide – which cannot explode – has been used.

It was not surgeons who took the next step – from diagnostic laparoscopy (looking inside the abdomen to see what there is to see) to therapeutic laparoscopy (looking inside the abdomen to do something) – but gynaecologists, because it is not only the liver that can be inspected with a laparoscope through the navel: there is also a perfect view of the womb and ovaries. All you have to do is tilt the operating table with the head downwards, so the intestines shift position from the lower to the upper abdomen. And because, unlike internists, gynaecologists were accustomed to performing operations, it only required a small step for them to conduct minor operations with the aid of a laparoscope. They started with laparoscopic sterilisation, which entailed tying off both fallopian tubes, and then went further, lancing cysts on the ovaries and removing ectopic pregnancies. As they got better at it, they performed increasingly complex procedures. German gynaecologist Kurt Semm removed uterine fibroids and was eventually able to remove a whole womb laparoscopically. In 1966, he marketed the first automatic insufflator, the CO2-Pneu-Automatik, which inflated the abdomen with carbon dioxide and kept it at a safe constant pressure. Semm also developed the first laparotrainer, a model in a box with which gynaecologists could learn how to perform laparoscopic operations.

In the Netherlands on 2 December 1975, Henk de Kok, a surgeon who learned laparoscopy from his brother Jef, a gynaecologist, performed the world's first laparoscopically assisted appendectomy at the hospital in the Dutch town of Gorinchem. With the laparoscope in one hand, he located the appendix and, with the other, he determined the location on the abdomen where he could make a minuscule incision through which he could extract the appendix, watching all the time through the laparoscope. His fellow surgeons thought the whole procedure scandalous.

Laparoscopy had never enjoyed much popularity among surgeons. Because you always had to hold the laparoscope with one hand, you only had one hand free to perform the procedure. Surgical applications of laparoscopy only really became possible with the advent of a completely new technology. In 1969, George Smith and Willard Boyle invented the charge-coupled device, better known as the CCD chip, which enables images to be digitalised and processed. The first CCD camera came on the market in 1982 and, within a few years, the latest models were small enough for a surgeon's assistant to hold the camera while the surgeon stood upright, watching the screen. Still, many surgeons were not convinced. The first video-assisted laparoscopic cholecystectomy – the removal of a gall bladder with a video camera and a television screen – was performed by Phillipe Mouret in Lyon in 1987. Mouret was in fact a gynaecologist, but the successful operation set many a surgeon's hands itching and, within a few years, laparoscopy had spread like wildfire.

The cholecystectomy became the most commonly performed laparoscopic operation in the world. It only requires three or four tiny incisions, altogether no bigger than four centimetres, while the incision for a classic gall bladder removal was longer than 15 centimetres. The public noticed the difference immediately, as the innovation was big news in the media. Patients experienced much less pain and no longer had to spend a week in hospital, but could go home the next day. It was the start of a trend that unleashed a genuine revolution. Minimal invasive surgery – performing the maximum surgical intervention with the smallest possible operational technique – became the magic word in twenty-first century surgical practice. It sounds so logical, but it was only possible as a result of complex high-tech developments.

Now, there is not a single organ in the abdomen that cannot be operated on laparoscopically. In 2001, French professor Jacques Marescaux built on Van der Heijden and Go's feat by performing a trans-Atlantic operation which – with an obvious sense of spectacle – he called Operation Lindberg. From New York, he controlled a robot in Strasbourg, performing a laparoscopic chole-cystectomy on a female patient nearly 4,000 miles away. More recently, without making an incision, Marescaux removed a gall bladder endoscopically through an opening in the vagina. Yet, despite surgeons' best efforts to showcase surgery as an innovative discipline, it is radiologists and cardiologists who have made the most spectacular progress in minimal invasive techniques in recent years. They can now replace a heart valve through a puncture in the groin, stop a bleeding spleen, remove a stone in the bile duct through the liver and treat a rupturing aortic aneurysm as if it is the easiest thing in the world, without the need for an operation at all.

As for non-surgical physicians, they stopped using diagnostic laparoscopy around the same time that surgical laparoscopy with a video camera began, but not because surgeons took it over from them. Other technologies had been developed, including ultrasound scans and computed tomography (CT) scanning, which give a much clearer image of the liver than laparoscopy.

Georg Kelling, the man who discovered laparoscopy, died at his home in 1945 during the bombing of Dresden. His body was never found.

18

Castration

The History of a Very Simple Operation: Adam, Eve and Farinelli

THE ANCIENT GREEK creation legend includes one of the most frequently performed surgical procedures in the history of humankind. Primal couple Uranus and Gaia, representing the sky and the earth, have children who are giants and Uranus, afraid that he will be usurped by one of his sons, casts them all into the underworld. But Uranus's fears prove true as, with the help of his mother, the Titan Cronos escapes, castrates his father and takes over the reins of power. For ten days, Uranus's genitals fall towards earth, finally plunging into the sea and giving birth to the goddess Aphrodite. Cronos is just as fearful of losing power as his father and devours all his own children, with the exception of Zeus, who escapes and later returns to kill his father. The three largest planets in our solar system are named after these three great gods: Uranus, Saturn (the Roman equivalent of Cronos) and Jupiter (the Roman equivalent of Zeus).

Castration also occurs in another creation legend – though in reverse form. The Egyptian god Osiris is cut into fourteen pieces by his angry brother Seth and spread all over the world. Isis, Osiris's wife, searches for the pieces and finds thirteen of them, which are then surgically reassembled. Isis becomes the Egyptian patroness of surgeons and Osiris is once again god enough to father a son by her, Horus. This is quite an accomplishment, since the missing fourteenth part of Osiris is his genitals. Horus eventually becomes the god of the sky and kills Seth.

It is not only the Egyptian creation legend that closely resembles the myth of Uranus and Cronos; the creation story in the Old Testament also has many similarities. As in the Greek version, the biblical story starts with the creation of a male and a female: Adam and a woman referred to in some interpretations as Lilith are created from the dust of the earth. In both legends, the man then undergoes an operation: Adam is anaesthetised and a rib is removed, while Uranus is castrated. From each of the removed body parts, a new woman is created – Aphrodite in the Greek version and Eve in the Bible. What is interesting about the biblical story, from a surgical perspective, is that the body part extracted from Adam is not, as with the Greeks and the Egyptians, the easy-to-remove genitals. Removing a rib was far too complex an operation for that time, in fact inconceivable, given the surgical dissection it requires. Furthermore, the Bible also tells us that the operation left a scar on Adam's body, yet, there is no scar on the side of a man's chest, and men have the same number of ribs as women: twenty-four.

But men are indeed born with scars. Two, to be precise, as biologist Scott Gilbert and biblical scholar Ziony Zevit pointed out in a fascinating article in 2001. The navel is a scar left over after the umbilical cord is discarded. The second scar is the perineal raphe, a vertical line exactly in the middle of the scrotum and the base of the penis, which is a remnant of the embryonic development of the male urethra. Nearly all other mammals have a bone beneath this line, known as the *baculum*, but men are among the few that do not. This is interesting because the Hebrew word *tzela*, used in the Bible, does mean 'rib' but also a support joist or buttress. With a little imagination *tzela* could refer to a different long, rigid bone, perhaps the *baculum*. Could this penis bone – that men do not have – be the 'rib' that was removed from Adam? Was it a castration after all, the resection of Adam's 'supporting buttress'?

As castration was apparently nothing out of the ordinary for the authors of these old myths, the operation must have very early origins. That is quite possible, since it is not a particularly complex procedure: you can easily cut, chop or strike off someone's genitals with even the simplest of tools – two rocks, for example. The castration of Cronos was recorded by Hesiod in the eighth century BC, but the story was already part of a much older tradition, and indeed there are references to castration in the Old Testament that state that men whose testicles have been crushed or cut out cannot enter heaven.

Initially, castration was a dangerous operation that served to punish or subjugate. In China and other parts of the Far East, it was applied as an alternative to execution for prisoners of war. The techniques were very cruel: in some cases the genitals were smeared with faeces and then bitten off by a dog. But even with less unhygienic methods, by simply cutting or chopping off everything hanging between the victim's legs, the chances of bleeding to death or developing gas gangrene were so high that the outcome differed little from a regular death sentence.

Yet, since at least 2,500 years ago, there must have been ways of castrating men without such a great risk, since not all of them underwent the operation as a form of punishment and it was often of great importance that it was successful. Persian kings received annual 'tax' payments from their provinces in the form of a set number of castrated young men from the most prominent families in the country. On the Greek island of Chios, a man called Panionios made his fortune performing castrations, a profession that was scandalous by Greek standards. This self-proclaimed surgeon would buy the most attractive slaves at the local market, castrate them and sell them at a high price on the mainland in Asia Minor. We do not know how he performed the operation, but he was clearly so successful at it that he could live well from the trade. One of his victims ended up as a eunuch at the Persian court, where he worked his way up to become a confidant of King Xerxes, which allowed him the opportunity to take revenge on the surgeon who robbed him of his manhood. He returned to Chios, where he forced Panionios to castrate his own four sons, who then had to return the favour on their father.

Eunuchs were a powerful and privileged group at the court and in the harems of kings, sultans and emperors in Asia, Arabia and Byzantium, the eastern Roman Empire. They were often influential men with high social status as diplomats, treasurers, civil servants or generals. Apparently, castrated men were appreciated for a number of positive qualities. They were seen as loyal, trustworthy, refined, astute, conciliatory and gifted with a talent for organisation. Traditionally, Mohammed's grave could only be guarded by eunuchs. Political power in China was even dominated by eunuchs for twenty-three dynasties and under the Ming emperors the country was ruled by 100,000 castrated public officials. The last surviving eunuch in the Forbidden City in China, Sun Yaoting, died in 1996.

In the severe version of castration, penis and scrotum were removed with one simple, decisive slash of the knife. An object – a goose feather, for example, or a special plug made of tin – was then inserted into the freshly transected urethra to keep it open. The operation was not performed by surgeons: in North Africa, slave traders did it themselves at the trading posts for black slaves from the Sudan destined for Ottoman sultans. They stemmed the flow of blood from the gaping wound with glowing hot desert sand. The blood poured out of the erectile tissues of the penis and the arteries of the testicles. If it did not stop in a day, the slave would bleed to death. If he survived until the next day, it was very likely that he would develop a life-threatening infection in the following weeks, when the wound should normally have been healing. It was a cruel selection process, determined more by coincidence and the cleanliness of the knife and bandages than the victim's strength and will to survive. But a slave who survived the ordeal was immediately worth several times the price he would have fetched otherwise.

In the Imperial City in Peking, the operation was performed by specialised castrators. Taking hold of the victim's genitals in their left hand and holding a curved knife behind them with their right hand, they asked the man (or, in the case of a minor, the father) whether the castration really should take place and, on hearing the word 'yes', they would pull the knife towards them, cutting the penis and scrotum off in one stroke. They then tended to the wound with oiled paper and allowed the victim to walk around the room for a couple of hours. The patient was not permitted to drink anything for three days, so as not to have to urinate. The castrator would preserve the genitals in vinegar in a labelled jar, to serve as a kind of lifelong guarantee for the imperial eunuch.

In the seventh century, Byzantine surgeon Paul of Aegina described two methods of castration that surgeons could apply to minimise the damage. At the same time, Aegina admitted that the operation went completely against the basic principle of surgery. Rather than restoring the natural order, it actually distorted it irrevocably. Moreover, castration was officially outlawed by the state and the church, and anyone performing it could be punished either by being castrated himself or by being eaten by wild animals. Nevertheless, writes Aegina, prominent figures frequently forced surgeons to perform castrations against their will, and the fact that Aegina describes this operation, which was so dangerous for both patient and surgeon, in his textbook probably means that too many castrations ended badly because they were not performed correctly.

According to Aegina, the first method was to castrate young

boys by putting them in a warm bath and slowly squeezing their testicles until you could no longer feel them. This was a risky undertaking – you could never be completely certain that the victim's libido might not manifest itself to some degree during adolescence. In the second method, the patient had to stand on a platform with his legs apart whereby a vertical incision would be made on both sides of the scrotum, as far as the testicles. The surgeon would then pull the scrotum down forcefully until the testicles popped out. He would then only have to peel away the shell surrounding them, remove them and tie off the spermatic chord.

These more selective castrations, which Aegina intended for real surgeons, thus spared the penis. A surgical clamp with the same intention has also been found on the bed of the River Thames, dating from the time of the Romans when the city was known as Londinium. It looks like a kind of elongated nutcracker, ornately decorated and with two serrated surfaces that come together when the forceps are closed. There is, however, a gap on the upper side. It may be a Roman castration clamp that can be placed on the scrotum without crushing the penis, allowing the scrotum to be easily removed with a knife. The clamp would then keep the blood vessels closed off to stem the bleeding.

Castrations were quite commonplace in the history of the Roman emperors. In the ninth century, Byzantine emperor Michael II not only overthrew his predecessor Leo V, but also had Leo's four sons castrated in order to bring the dynasty of his rival to an end. One of them died from loss of blood, another was allegedly struck dumb. Two Roman emperors fell in love with men and had them castrated by a surgeon so that they could marry them: Nero with a man called Sporus and Heliogabalus with a charioteer called Hierocles.

These three different methods produced three different kinds of eunuch. The Byzantine Romans called them *castrati* (no penis or scrotum), *spadones* (without testicles but with a penis) and *thlibiae* (with crushed testicles). By practising castration on a large scale, the Byzantines and the Chinese created a separate social class of eunuchs within their societies. The eunuch class was intended to act as a safe but efficient buffer between the male ruler and all other men with ambitions in the kingdom, and between the ruler and his women. But it was not only about politics and securing power and lineage. By surrounding themselves with a large group of eunuchs, the leaders also preserved the mystery of the court. In Christian Byzantium, it represented a literal extension of the biblical creation legend of Adam and Eve. That story already described an operation – the surgical removal of one of Adam's ribs to create the female sex – but the Byzantines went a step further and created another sex from Adam, again with an operation: a sexless gender in between male and female. These were the angels, who had undeniably male characteristics, but never grew beards. In that sense, they were consistent in the practice of their faith: it was not only the Christian emperors who surrounded themselves with hosts of sexless beings; their God did the same.

A castration is a primal operation – simple, dangerous and with serious consequences. Anyone could do it: a father could castrate his son, a victor his vanquished enemy, a man could even castrate himself. After all, ultimately it was simply a matter of cutting off an appendage, just as Abraham had removed his own foreskin. It was as easy as an executioner chopping off hands, ears or a nose, or cutting out a tongue. Such operations require three decisive surgical actions: localisation (deciding where and what to cut), incision (making the cut) and haemostasis (stopping the bleeding). By comparison, even a simple modern-day operation like removing a small fatty lump requires at least six surgical actions: localisation, incision, dissection (dividing, searching and separating) resection (removing or extracting), haemostasis and suture, (closing

Gills

As our bodies develop in the womb, the embryo again passes through the same phases that we experienced in our evolution from single-cell beings to humans. Sometime in the first few weeks of the pregnancy, we are briefly creatures with gills, like fish, five on each side of our head. The gills then close up again and grow together, eventually forming the face and neck. If something goes wrong at this stage in the development of the embryo, the child is left with a defect, a scar or a cleft lip or palate. These are congenital disorders that can only be corrected surgically. A cleft palate is known medically as palatoschisis, a cleft lip (or harelip) as cheiloschisis and a cleft lip, jaw and palate, which can extend as far as the eye socket and eyelid, as cheilognathopalatoschisis. Similar problems can also occur elsewhere, such as in spina bifida (when the tube of the embryonic nervous system does not close completely) or hypospadias (incomplete development of the urethra). Structures evolve from the five gill arches that you would not expect to be related to either fish or gills. The first arch gives rise to the middle ear – two of the three middle ear bones (auditory ossicles) and the Eustachian tube. The second forms the third auditory ossicle (the stapes), the hyoid bone (tongue bone) and the pharyngeal tonsil (adenoid). The parathyroid glands and the thymus are formed from the third and fourth gill arch and the fourth and fifth develop into the thyroid gland and the larynx (with the vocal cords). So anyone who thinks we were created from anything else is simply wrong – we started off as fish.

the wound). More complex operations (such as removing a rib) entail more steps. Highly complex procedures like removing the oesophagus, rectum or pancreas require around a hundred decisive surgical actions to bring them to a successful conclusion.

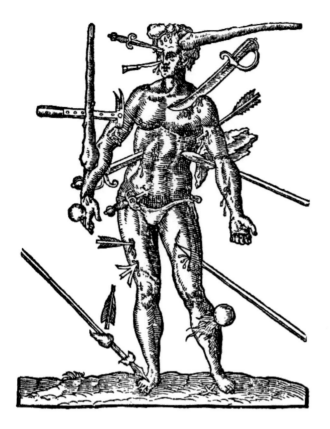

Woodcut print from the 1594 book *Opera Chirurgica* (*Surgical Works*) by French army surgeon Ambroise Paré, showing various war injuries one could encounter as an army surgeon. (Ambroise Paré, 1594)

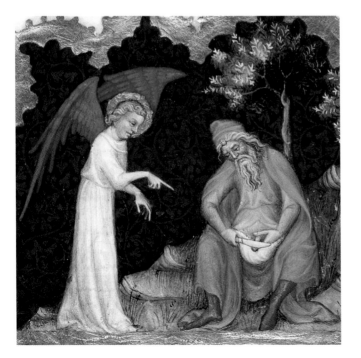

In the Old Testament, patriarch Abraham performs a surgical operation on himself, trying to cure what might have been a disease of the object he cut away: the foreskin of his penis. The relief must have been great, as he did not hesitate to perform the same operation on all males of his household. (Maître de la Bible de Jean de Sy, ca. 1355–1357)

The colon, or large intestine, is situated not far below the skin. A colostomy can be performed by bringing out the colon through the skin. The suffix '-stomy' means opening. (Blausen.com staff (2014). "Medical gallery of Blausen Medical 2014". *WikiJournal of Medicine* 1 (2). DOI:10.15347/wjm/2014.010. ISSN 2002-4436.)

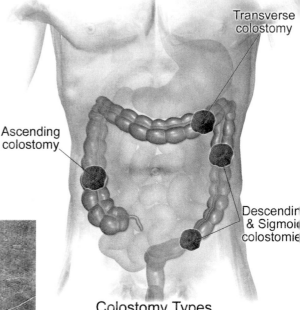

Transverse colostomy

Ascending colostomy

Descendir & Sigmoie colostomie

Colostomy Types

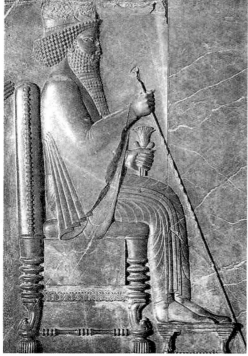

ABOVE: When Darius the Great seized power in 521 BC, he became both king of the Persian Empire and pharaoh of Egypt. None of the many images of him, including this relief carving in Persepolis, show his alleged physical handicap from a complex ankle fracture. (Frank Haf)

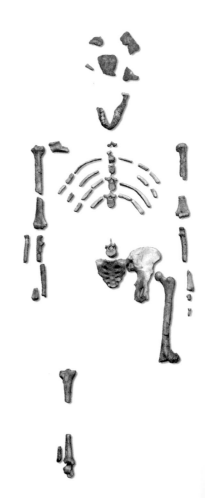

RIGHT: These remains of the skeleton of a female human ancestor, nicknamed 'Lucy', were found in 1974. Lucy was an *Australopithecus afarensis,* an extinct species of the family of hominids, the scientific name for human-like animals. (Vincent Mourre, 2007)

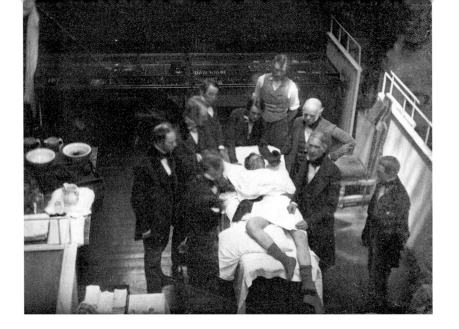

ABOVE: Reenactment of the first operation performed using ether anesthesia, shortly after the actual operation took place on 16 October 1846 at the Massachusetts General Hospital in Boston. (Southworth & Hawes, 1846)

BELOW: Albert Einstein visited New York for the first time on 2 April 1921, arriving with his wife, Elsa, on the steamship *Rotterdam*. It was later in New York that he met a fellow countryman, German surgeon Rudolph Nissen, who operated on his – ultimately fatal – abdominal aneurysm in 1948. (Underwood & Underwood, 1921)

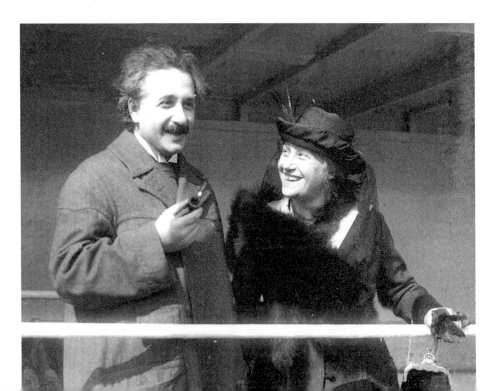

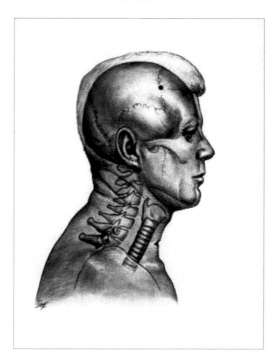

ABOVE: President John F. Kennedy was shot at three times on 22 November 1963. The first bullet missed its target, but the other two were deadly: the second one hit the president in his back and pierced his windpipe, and the third damaged parts of his skull and brain. This medical drawing by Ida Dox depicts the windpipe behind the bullet exit wound in the front of the neck. (Warren Commission exhibit F-58, 1963)

BELOW: Lee Harvey Oswald's arrest card in Dallas, 23 November 1963. One day after his arrest for assassinating President John F. Kennedy, he was assassinated himself, shot in the upper part of his abdomen by Jack Ruby. He did not survive the attack, despite a heroic operation that involved several vital organs in his abdomen and his heart. (Heritage Auction Gallery, Warren Commission, 1963)

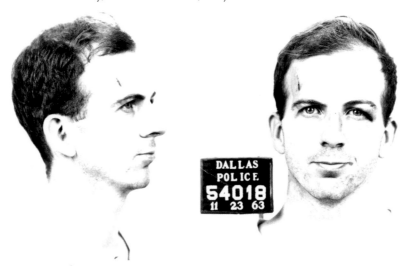

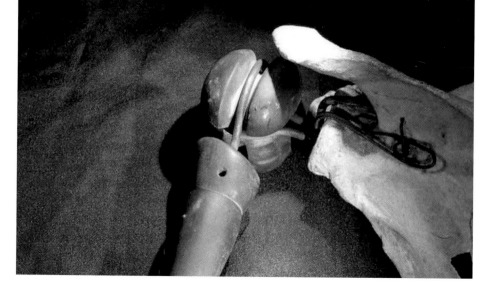

ABOVE: No human body would ever tolerate this nineteenth-century artificial shoulder made of platinum and rubber, especially not in the presence of a fierce infection like tuberculosis of the bone. Yet French surgeon Jules-Émile Péan implanted this contraption in 1893 in a patient suffering from consumption. It had to be removed two years later. The antique prosthesis is now located in Washington DC. (Alan Hawk, 1993)

BELOW: Painting of famous French surgeon Jules-Émile Péan, before the operation, by Henri Gervex (Paris 1887). The surgeon is portrayed as a hero about to save a life. (Gebbie & Husson Co., 1889)

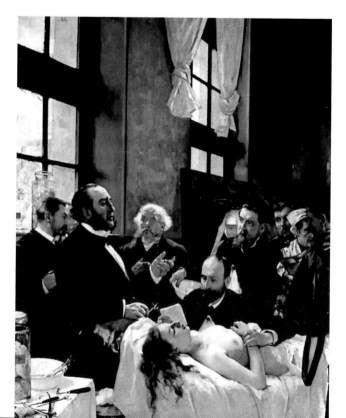

In the late twentieth century, Austrian surgeon Theodor Billroth was practically a god to doctors and surgeons. The characters depicted in this 1890 painting by Adalbert Seligmann focus on Billroth as the central figure. (Adalbert Seligmann, 1890)

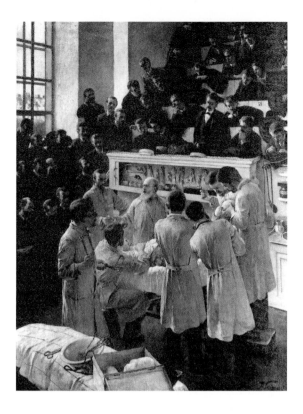

Surgeon William Halsted operating at Johns Hopkins Hospital in Baltimore, Maryland, in 1904. Halsted was the first to use rubber gloves during an operation, mainly to protect the skin against the disinfecting chemicals. (Wellcome Collection)

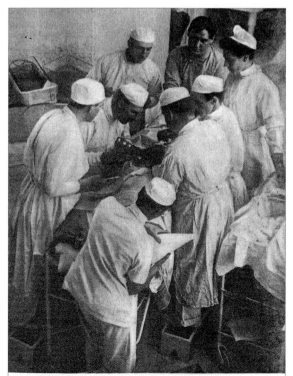

Dr. Halsted's First Operation in the New Surgical Amphitheatre in 1904

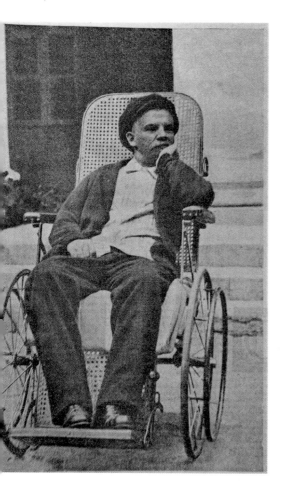

Although Vladimir Ilyich Uljanov – or Lenin, as he was more commonly known – never smoked, he suffered from a series of strokes at a relatively young age. In this photograph of Lenin recovering from his third stroke, taken on 28 August 1923, the paralysis of his right arm is clearly visible. (M. I. Ulyanova, 1923)

ithout artificial light, no
vity of the body could be
spected that was farther
vay than the reach of a
ctor's finger. For centu-
es, these were inspected
ith the light of the sun or
andle. The first organ
be reached by artificial
ght was the stomach, with
netal tube the size of a
oman sword that had to be
vallowed in its entirety. On
e tip there was a small elec-
c lightbulb, illuminating
e organ from the inside.
Vikimedia Commons)

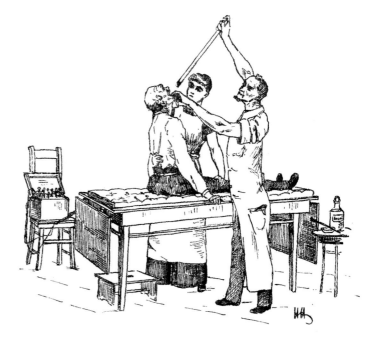

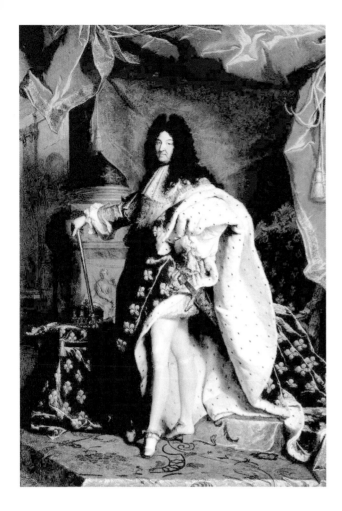

King Louis XIV was France's magnificent seventeenth-century monarch known as the Sun King, but this didn't prevent him from falling victim to a painful anal fistula. The fact that he dared to undergo an operation – and survived – would have given the reputation of his surgeon's profession a tremendous boost. (Louis XIV Collection, 1701)

The electric eel of Amsterdam's Artis Zoo during his operation to examine a tumor in 2013. The tube in his mouth supplied fresh oxygenated water containing anesthesia, so that the operation could be performed without electric shock hazard. (From Arnold van de Laar's personal collection.)

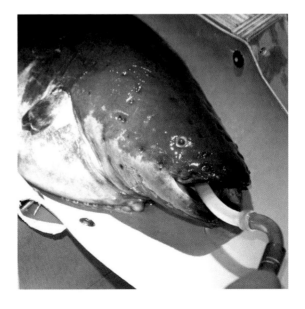

And yet, the greatest difference between common-or-garden operations, like castration, and a real surgical procedure is not the number of actions required. It is dissection.

Dissection, a Latin word meaning 'cut away from each other', embraces all surgical techniques to search for and find the right surgical plane. Surgery is all about planes. Our bodies are made up of a large number of anatomical layers that remain intact from the very beginning – during the development of the embryo – through to adulthood, but can be separated from each other by dissection. The important thing is to recognise the different layers, to stay in the right plane between them and to know what important structures are to be found in which layer. Dissection is thus the practice of separating different layers and structures, recognising them and cutting through them, while leaving the rest intact.

With operations involving only one incision, dissection is not necessary. But the second method proposed by Paul of Aegina, peeling the testicles out of their shells and then removing them, required a form of dissection – a testicle is surrounded by no fewer than four layers – and you needed a surgeon with experience and skill to do that. But given the enormous number of castrations that took place throughout the history of humankind, most of which were not carried out by skilled surgeons, there must still have been hordes of surgeons performing the procedure. And those surgeons had the blood of many innocent young men on their hands – literally and figuratively.

A castration has major consequences, depending on the technique used and the age at which the production of the male hormone testosterone is interrupted. Testosterone is produced by the testicles from puberty onwards. First of all, cutting off a penis caused two opposing problems in the urethra, or what was left of it. The scar had the tendency to close up the hole in the urethra, making it increasingly difficult to urinate, but the operation also affected the working of the sphincter, so that the patient could no longer retain his urine. This combination of incontinence and narrowing of the urethra meant that eunuchs lost urine during the whole day, drip by drip. In both China and the Ottoman Empire, they used a metal rod with a string or a knob on the end, which they inserted in the urethra to close it off and also to stop the opening from narrowing. The shift in the eunuchs' hormone balance made their bones grow more rapidly, so that they suffered osteoporosis at a young age, which caused spontaneous compression of the vertebrae. They lost body hair, their breast tissue increased and their voices became weaker. All in all, a eunuch could be recognised by the sour smell of urine, a heavy build with a typically crooked posture, a smooth face and a sing-song voice. This bizarre operation also had its advantages: eunuchs tended to live longer than average, though that may have been more a consequence of their protected and privileged position in society, where they enjoyed better living conditions than their contemporaries.

The fact that castration can prevent young boys' singing voices from breaking in puberty has led to a fascinating chapter in the history of surgical emasculation. In the eighteenth century, *castrati* – castrated male sopranos – were an absolute sensation in Europe. They were the megastars of Italian opera, whose soprano voices set many a female heart beating faster. The biggest idol of all was Carlo Broschi, known in his young years as *il ragazzo* ('the young boy') and later under his stage name as Farinelli. He was castrated as a child because he had such a beautiful voice. He sang in Rome, Vienna, London, Paris and Madrid and at the pinnacle of his career his voice range extended from the A below the middle C to the D above the high C. In Spain, his voice had such a soothing effect on the king, who was tormented by depressive melancholy, that he offered Farinelli a position as a minister. He spent many years of his life, like the Chinese nightingale in Hans

Christian Andersen's fairy tale, singing to the king evening after evening, and died in Italy in 1782 at the age of seventy-eight.

Farinelli did not, of course, owe his success purely to being castrated: he had been born with a wonderful voice. It is alarming to think how many hundreds or thousands of young boys with ambitious parents were castrated in those times in the hope of achieving similar success, but who proved not to have the required talent.

Castrati were immensely popular in the baroque era, but had been a common feature of opera and religious music long before, and would remain so long after. For many centuries, women were forbidden to perform in public, and *castrati* played the female roles in opera. As women were also not permitted to sing in church, *castrati* were illustrious members of the papal choir in the Sistine Chapel in Rome and so castration for the purpose of preserving the voice was not banned in Italy until 1870 – though in the Vatican castration continued for more than thirty years after that and *castrati* were still singing in the papal choir until the beginning of the twentieth century. One of them was Alessandro Moreschi, the first and last *castrato* whose voice has been preserved on a gramophone record. Moreschi died in 1922.

The libido also becomes weaker after castration, which was of course usually the intention. For that reason, castration was used until not so long ago to 'cure' people of what was considered to be perverted sexual preferences. A well-known victim was Alan Turing, who cracked the Enigma code and invented the computer during the Second World War, but was sentenced to undergo chemical castration by a judge in 1952 because of his homosexuality.

Castrations are still performed today. Every year, the testicles of tens of thousands of men worldwide are surgically removed as part of the treatment for prostate cancer. The male hormone testosterone stimulates the growth of prostate cancer cells and stopping production of the hormone through castration can help slow down the spread of the cancer. Unlike all the other reasons used in history to castrate men, the treatment of cancer is of course a good reason to consider undergoing such a severe operation. Furthermore, prostate cancer – and therefore the need to perform a castration to combat it – usually occurs at a later age, after the patient has passed the reproductive phase of his life.

19

Lung Cancer

Thoracotomy at Home: King George VI

O N 23 SEPTEMBER 1951, after many days of preparation, English surgeon Clement Price-Thomas gave up his free Sunday morning to perform an operation that was, for a number of reasons, remarkable. Not only because it was a pneumectomy, an operation to remove an entire lung, or because the patient was the British King George VI – father of the current queen, Elizabeth II. It was also notable for the fact that the venue was the patient's own home: an operating room, just like the one the surgeon usually worked in at Westminster Hospital, had been set up in one of the rooms at Buckingham Palace.

George VI had lung cancer. In June of that year, he had withdrawn from public life, officially stating that it was due to a bout of flu. But the real diagnosis was not specified by name; the press release spoke only of 'structural changes' in the lung. In the 2010 film *The King's Speech*, it is suggested that George VI's doctors advised him to inhale cigarette smoke to help relieve his stutter. Inhaling smoke was something of a fad that had originated around the beginning of the century. For a long time – and thus still in 1951 – it was not considered to be harmful. Both the king and his surgeon were chain-smokers and there is a good chance that they even had a quick cigarette before the operation.

Tobacco first came to Europe in the sixteenth century. It was chewed, sniffed or smoked in a pipe. It was a very successful product and soon became a part of daily life. It even found its way into surgical terminology. The triangular hollow on the back of the hand that appears at the base of the thumb when you spread your fingers is known as the anatomical snuffbox, and is important in traumatology because pain in the snuffbox when pressure is applied can mean that the underlying bone, the scaphoid, is broken. Dutch surgeons must have been particularly fond of tobacco. A surgical suture placed around a structure or opening in the body to pull it closed is known throughout the world as a 'purse string', but in the Netherlands it is called a 'tobacco-pouch suture'. Calcified hardening of the small, elongated arteries in the lower leg as the result of diabetes is known very appropriately in Dutch as 'pipe-stem hardening', after the long, slim pipes made of white clay used to smoke tobacco.

Cigars became popular in the nineteenth century, while cigarettes became widespread in the twentieth century. Until then, tobacco consumed by sniffing, chewing or smoking a pipe or cigar never penetrated further into the body than the mouth, nose or throat. For four centuries, this led to many forms of cancer, but they were limited to the upper parts of the airways. Chewing tobacco, for example, caused cancer of the lips and tongue, and smoking cigars, of the throat. In the seventeenth century, there are records of several cases of tumours in the mouth, for example in the books of the Amsterdam chirurgeons Job van Meekren and Nicolaes Tulp, and a specific case of 'bastard flesh (cancer) and decay of the palate, fortuitously removed with the knife and glowing branding irons' recorded by Frederik Ruysch. Sigmund Freud, the psychoanalyst who was known for always having a cigar in his mouth, died of mouth cancer in 1939. The much-loved German emperor Friedrich III, also a cigar-smoker, died a miserable death of throat cancer in 1888. But lung cancer had always been a rarity, almost non-existent. Cancer from other parts of the body would sometimes spread to the lungs, but primary lung tumours, that is originating in the lung tissue itself, hardly occurred. A thesis published in 1912 listed all cases of lung cancer in the world recorded up to that date. There were less than 400. And then suddenly, out of nowhere, the figures for lung cancer increased explosively between 1920 and 1960 and it became a 'normal' disease. Lung cancer eventually became the most common cause of death from cancer, with more than a million fatalities worldwide every year. Initially, no one had any idea where these tumours came from.

Until modern times, cancer was rare. This is perhaps because people died earlier from other causes, whereas cancer typically develops at a later age. The reason why cells that have functioned perfectly normally suddenly turn malignant has been clarified for several forms of cancer by developments in genetics. A clear external cause can only be identified in limited types of cancer. John Hill was the first to find a clear link, in 1761, between long-term use of snuff and cancer of the nasal cavity. In 1775, Percival Pott noted that the strikingly high incidence of scrotal cancer among English chimney sweeps must have something to do with soot. Later, a connection was also found between bladder cancer and working with solvents used in paint, but the cause of the explosive number of cases of lung cancer long remained a mystery. A link with cigarette smoking had already been suspected in the 1930s, but it was not demonstrated conclusively until a number of large-scale patient surveys were conducted in the 1950s. Even then, it took a depressingly long time for the message to get through to doctors and surgeons. No one wanted to believe it.

With hindsight, graphs show very clearly that the increase in lung cancer ran completely parallel to the rise in cigarette consumption, with a delay of around twenty years. The full scale of the damage from inhaling smoke only became visible after the cigarette had become an integral part of modern culture and the daily life of millions of people. And it wasn't just movie stars and musicians: up to the 1970s it was still perfectly normal for a doctor to smoke in his consulting room, or for children to treat their schoolmates to sweet cigarettes on their birthdays, or their teachers to real ones.

Smoking can also give rise to other kinds of cancer in the body, such as breast cancer, pancreatic cancer and skin cancer. In addition, it can cause lung emphysema and chronic bronchitis, and is the main cause of cardiovascular diseases. There is no profession (other than that of cigarette manufacturer) that benefits as much from this bad habit as surgery. Most patients of vascular surgeons are smokers (hardened arteries caused by smoking lead to intermittent claudication, strokes and impotence), as are those of cardiac surgeons (smoking-related hardening of the arteries causes heart attacks) and of oncological surgeons (smoking causes a wide variety of cancers). Pulmonary (lung) surgery in particular has become prominent thanks to the cigarette.

Lung surgery is an exceptional challenge, because the lung is an exceptional organ. The lungs are located, separately from each other, in a hermetically sealed part of the thorax (chest). To get at the lungs, the chest has to be cut open between two ribs. This operation is known as a thoracotomy, an incision in the chest. For that reason pulmonary surgery is also known as thoracic surgery.

The distance between two ribs is less than two centimetres. To perform an operation on the lung in the chest cavity, that small gap has to be widened far enough to get both hands through. That is why, during a thoracotomy, the patient lies on his side and the operating table is tilted downwards at both ends so that the shoulders and the pelvis are lower than the ribs. This is known as 'breaking' the table. The skin is then cut open along the line of a rib. A number of muscles of the back, the chest and the shoulder girdle then have to be moved or loosened to make the ribs visible. The chest cavity is usually opened between the fourth and fifth ribs using a special rib spreader inserted between the two ribs, which are slowly pushed apart until the gap is around twenty centimetres wide. The break in the operating table helps to open the chest cavity. You can then see the lung in the chest cavity and, on the left, the pericardium, the sac holding the beating heart.

Breathing exposes our lungs permanently to the outside world. As a result they contain large quantities of external material and pathogens, which affects their appearance. A young lung is light-pink and soft, while the lung of an old smoker is black, hard and grainy. It also means that operating on the lungs makes infections more likely. The lungs are unique organs in the body that have their own circulatory system. They are supplied with blood from the right half of the heart, rather than the left and the blood pressure in the arteries in the lungs is five times lower than in the rest of the body. That is necessary because the delicate alveoli in the lungs could not withstand the high blood pressure. The arteries of the lung consequently have much thinner walls, making them more fragile and meaning that surgical sutures can easily rip.

The airways, too, are not easy to deal with. These rigid tubes are strong enough to resist the permanent fluctuations caused by inhaling and exhaling and are kept open by rings of cartilage, which makes it difficult to close a bronchus (airway) with a suture. To make sure the stitches were airtight, the thread used to be soaked in paraffin. Today, stapling machines are used. Even so, considerable pressure can be exerted on these sutures when patients cough following their operations. The lungs are thus like sponges that contain air. They cannot keep themselves open but are sucked open by negative pressure in the chest and so after an operation that negative pressure has to be restored by inserting a chest tube, a plastic suction tube, between the ribs. Removing a whole lung (a pneumectomy), however, leaves a hollow space where the pressure should not be negative. The empty chest cavity has to gradually fill itself with fluid and then scar tissue. In the meantime, infections or an air leak can lead to serious complications.

Smoking

Nothing is as unhealthy as smoking. Smokers find that difficult to accept. 'You can also be killed crossing the road' is one of the most often-heard excuses when they visit the doctor. That may be so, but the 28,000 Europeans who were killed on the roads in 2015 are a drop in the ocean compared with the 700,000 who died that year from smoking. About a quarter of all people in the world smoke. Half of them will die from their habit and half of those even before they reach retirement age. 'My grandpa has smoked for his whole life and he hasn't got lung cancer' is the second most common excuse. That may also be true, but smoking causes many more health problems than lung cancer alone. There is a good chance that, after smoking all his life, grandpa will die of a stroke, a heart attack, emphysema, pancreatic cancer, an aortic aneurysm or gangrene in the legs – all diseases caused by smoking. Impotence, facial wrinkles, gum infections and stomach ulcers will not kill you, but they are all smoking-related. Chronic infections of the middle ear among children almost always occur only if the parents smoke. Smoking during pregnancy stunts the child's development. And, to top it all, smoking is an important risk factor in post-operative complications, no matter what they are. So if you have to undergo an operation and are afraid of the risks, don't light up a cigarette to deal with the stress. Stop smoking.

Another problem with removing a whole lung is that, from one moment to the next, the entire circulatory system has to flow through only one lung, rather than two. That doubles the resistance of the blood flow, suddenly increasing the load on the heart. The first successful resection of a whole lung was not performed until 1931 when Rudolf Nissen (the surgeon who would later operate on Einstein) operated on an eleven-year-old girl. At the first attempt, she suffered a cardiac arrest but, on a second attempt, her heart proved able to withstand the sudden changes in circulation. Before this heroic feat, resections had been performed on part of a lung (in cases of tuberculosis, for example) but they were less risky, because there was always sufficient lung tissue left to fill up the chest cavity.

Two years after Nissen, in 1933, the first successful pneumectomy for lung cancer was performed in St Louis in the United States. The surgeon, Evarts Graham, would later play a different role in the cigarette story. Graham was also a smoker, as was his patient, Dr James Gilmore, a forty-eight-year-old gynaecologist. Cancer had been diagnosed in Gilmore's left lung by means of a bronchoscopy, an internal examination of the airways, which, at that time, was performed by pushing a straight rigid tube through the patient's mouth and down the windpipe. Gilmore weighed up his chances: they didn't seem promising. Until then, Graham had only performed a pneumectomy on test animals. The operation was therefore a dangerous experiment, but dying from lung cancer would be very unpleasant. Before the operation, Gilmore got his dentist to remove his gold fillings and used them to buy a plot in a cemetery. The evening before the operation, a resident physician came to Gilmore's bedside and urged him to leave the hospital. But the operation went ahead. The thoracotomy went surprisingly well and the tumour was clearly visible. Graham applied a clamp to the artery feeding the lung for a minute and a half to see if the heart could deal with the extra pressure. There were no serious problems, so he tied off the artery, then the veins and the primary bronchus. The lung was now free.

Graham was alarmed at the enormous space left after he had lifted the large organ out of the chest cavity and so he spent a further hour removing a number of ribs in order to somewhat collapse the ribcage. That strangely distorted the shape of the chest, but did reduce the size of the cavity. Gilmore stayed in the hospital for seventy-five days and had to be operated on again twice because of infections. Nevertheless he made a full recovery and resumed his work as a gynaecologist without problems, but with only one lung.

Gilmore was incredibly lucky. Lung cancer is a lethal disease that has usually spread by the time it is diagnosed. Even if treatment is possible, there is still a very high probability that the cancer will recur in the years following. In the case of Dr Gilmore, the lung cancer was apparently discovered at an early stage, because it never returned after the operation. He lived for another forty years (and carried on smoking until his death).

The operation on King George VI in Buckingham Palace also went well, though little is known about how the king responded to the operation or his recovery. His Christmas message on the radio that year was apparently weak and compiled from various fragments recorded in advance. The king only lived for another four months after this pneumectomy, dying of a cardiac arrest in his sleep. He was fifty-six years old. His daughter and successor, Elizabeth, was on a visit to Kenya. She came home to be the Queen of England.

The resection of his right lung was not the only operation George VI underwent in his life. In 1917, he had been operated on for a peptic ulcer (stomach ulcer) and in 1949 on hardened arteries (arteriosclerosis) in the legs. All three diseases – arteriosclerosis, a peptic ulcer and lung cancer – are smoking related. As is, of course, a cardiac arrest, which the king ultimately died of.

Indeed, smoking-related illnesses are not uncommon for the

royal family. George VI's father George V and his grandfather Edward VII were both heavy smokers as well and both died of emphysema. They, too, had been operated on at the palace, Edward for appendicitis on the day of his coronation and George for an abscess next to a lung. George VI's second daughter, Princess Margaret, smoked from her teenage years and contracted lung cancer in 1985, and she was successfully operated on. She died in 2002 of a stroke, also smoking-related despite the fact that she had stopped some years previously. The mother of George VI, Queen Mary, died in 1953, a year after her son, of the same disease: lung cancer. George's brother Edward also smoked. As mentioned earlier, he was operated on in Houston in December 1964 by surgeon Michael DeBakey for an aortic aneurysm and was later diagnosed with throat cancer – needless to say, both are also smoking-related.

Royal surgeon Clement Price-Thomas was knighted by his own patient. The surgeon carried on smoking – and contracted lung cancer. He was operated on by doctors Charles Drew and Peter Jones, who had assisted him at Buckingham Palace and were now surgeons themselves. They performed a lobectomy, removal of part of the lung, and with success: Price-Thomas lived on for many years in good health.

Surgeon Evarts Graham in St Louis thought the idea that lung cancer was related to smoking ridiculous. To prove that he was right, he studied 684 of his lung cancer patients but he discovered the complete opposite. This groundbreaking study, published in 1950, showed an irrefutable link between cancer and smoking, demonstrating for the first time that smoking has a carcinogenic effect. In the years that followed, however, sales of cigarettes continued to rise. For Graham, who had smoked his whole life, the realisation of the harm he was doing to his body came too late. He contracted lung cancer himself and died in 1957. His patient James Gilmore visited him as he lay on his deathbed.

Despite his one lung and deformed chest, Gilmore was as fit as a fiddle. The annual turnover of tobacco manufacturer Philip Morris in that year was 20 billion dollars.

20

Placebo

The Fifth Man on the Moon: Alan Shepard

I N THE MIDDLE Ages, anyone who wanted to add a little lustre to their funeral could hire a group of monks to come and sing Psalm 114. The final sentence in particular gave extra drama to the final farewell: 'I shall please the Lord in the land of the living'. It wasn't cheap, but it assured you a long-remembered send-off. The singers themselves, of course, had nothing to do with the deceased. Their lamenting was all pretence. They were essentially fake-mourners, commercial clerics who were referred to mockingly by the word they sang most dramatically of all: *placebo*, Latin for 'I shall please'.

A placebo is something that is not actually active in treating a medical problem, but, if presented as such, can cause a beneficial effect. A well-known example is homeopathy, in which mixtures containing no active ingredients are prescribed for certain ailments or diseases. Placebos do not always have to be potions or pills. Well-intended acupuncture needles or osteopathic manipulations are forms of 'treatment' that, in reality, are not that at all. Therefore a placebo itself does not have any beneficial effect, but believing in it does. The mechanism driving that effect is purely psychological and contains elements of expectation, recognition, attention and suggestion. For some time, it was assumed that placebos had a valuable role to play in medical treatment, but this has since been proved to be untrue and that their functional impact is very limited. The result of a placebo treatment can thus often be beneficial, but is mostly not useful. In homeopathy, for example, doctor and patient often maintain a long-term relationship. It does not end in a cure, but is perpetuated by the repeated prescription of remedies that do not work, allowing the symptoms to persist. The great disadvantage of this is that the patient becomes increasingly labelled as a chronic sufferer, making the step back to a normal, healthy life more and more difficult.

The placebo effect is nothing new. The walls of the Lady Chapel in the Cathedral of St John in the Dutch city of 's-Hertogenbosch are adorned with votive offerings in silver or wax, in the form of small legs or arms, donated by grateful patients who have been cured of their diseases and ailments throughout the centuries. In the cave at Lourdes, where the Virgin Mary is alleged to have appeared to a young shepherdess, hang the crutches of cripples who found they could walk again.

The placebo effect conforms to a number of rules. First, the patient must be convinced that it will work. He or she must therefore not know (or want to know) that the treatment is fake. The effect will be stronger if the person administering it also believes that it will work. And it will work even better if administered with a certain degree of pomp and circumstance. A surgical procedure therefore has all the potential to be a powerful placebo. After all, neither patient nor surgeon would dare to run the risk of complications if they are not convinced that the operation will be a success. And, of course, surgery is quite a lot more dramatic than a pill or a drink.

The placebo effect is weaker among patients who derive considerable satisfaction from their bad health, for example people who thrive on the sympathy and attention they receive because of it. Conversely, the effect can be reinforced among patients who would benefit more than average from a successful treatment.

No one could ever have expected to gain so much from being cured as Alan B. Shepard when he consented to an operation in

1969. Shepard was lined up to undergo the ultimate adventure when he contracted a disease that threatened to make him completely unsuitable for a once-in-a-lifetime opportunity.

Shepard was thirty-seven when he became the first American to go into space. Although the flight lasted only fifteen minutes and his Mercury spacecraft followed a sub-orbital ballistic trajectory, Shepard was briefly a hero, at least in the United States. The mission had actually been just too late – twenty-three days earlier, the Russian Yuri Gagarin had become the first man in space and had orbited the earth for more than an hour – but Shepard's flight heralded the start of a much greater adventure: the journey to the Moon.

The Mercury missions were followed by the Gemini capsule and the Apollo project. Of the original seven Mercury astronauts, six played a role in the long series of missions that led to the Moon. John Glenn was the first American to orbit the earth, Scott Carpenter the second, Gordon Cooper was the first to spend a night in space, Gus Grissom the first to be killed during the lunar space programme, Walter Schirra the first to fly the Apollo and Deke Slayton the last.

Only Alan Shepard came no further. He was found unfit for medical reasons, as he was suffering from a form of Ménière's disease – idiopathic vestibular dysfunction, to be precise. Idiopathic means a disease without a clearly identifiable cause, and vestibular refers to the system in the inner ear that regulates our sense of balance. The disease causes spontaneous attacks of vertigo and tinnitus. Shepard could suddenly hear a buzzing sound in his left ear and would feel as if everything around him was spinning. This was followed by nausea, like seasickness, which was sometimes so bad that he had to vomit. He took a medicine called Diamox to combat the disease, believed to be caused by excess pressure of the endolymph fluid in the semicircular canals of the vestibular system in the inner ear. Diamox is a diuretic, a pill that promotes the excretion of water, which could have reduced the excess fluid in the inner ear, but unfortunately in Shepard's case it did not work. An unexpected attack of dizziness, vomiting and loss of balance could naturally be catastrophic to a test pilot who spends hundreds of hours in a jet plane. Or a space rocket.

Shepard was grounded and given a desk job at NASA, where he soon gained a reputation as the most bad-tempered official at the agency. As his colleagues made one space voyage after another, Shepard heard of a new, experimental operation that might be able to help him. The surgeon was fully convinced that it would work.

A few months before Neil Armstrong flew to the Moon, Shepard was operated on in Los Angeles by ear, nose and throat specialist William House. House inserted a tiny silicone tube through the petrous part of the temporal bone and into the inner ear to drain the excess endolymph fluid. This procedure is known as an endolymphatic shunt. Theoretically, this would reduce the pressure in the vestibular system. The details of this procedure are not very relevant here. What is important is that, after the operation, Shepard no longer suffered from his attacks.

NASA's doctors examined him and passed him for flight duty. In May 1969, aged forty-five, Shepard was reinstated as an astronaut and began training for the Apollo 13 mission. But because of his age, he needed longer to get fit for the voyage to the Moon and so he was moved back one mission. A lucky decision for him, with hindsight, as Apollo 13 experienced trouble during the flight (the immortal words 'Houston, we have a problem' were uttered by the astronaut who replaced him). But, on 31 January 1971, Alan B. Shepard finally got his flight to the Moon. As commander of Apollo 14, he was even responsible for the most demanding task of the whole mission: landing the lunar module Antares on the Fra Mauro Highlands on 5 February 1971. It would prove to be the most precise lunar landing of all the Apollo missions.

It was essential for the astronauts to perform this manoeuvre standing up, so that they could feel the movements of the module in the Moon's weak gravity with their own sense of balance. Just how remarkable it was that Shepard did this faultlessly emerged more than ten years later, when it was shown that the outcome of the endolymphatic shunt was based entirely on a placebo effect.

This was demonstrated by the following experiment: A group of patients with Ménière's disease were tested for an operation. Lots were drawn. An important part of the endolymphatic shunt procedure is the removal of the mastoid bone, the knob of bone that you can feel as a hard lump behind your ear, another part of the temporal bone. Removing it gives the surgeon access to the minuscule cavities of the inner ear. Half of the patients in the group underwent a full endolymphatic shunt operation, while the others only had their mastoid bones removed – a procedure that would have no effect on their symptoms. It was not possible to see or feel on the outside who had undergone which procedure. They were then all tested over a period of three years with neither the patients nor the doctors who tested them knowing who had had which operation. This is known as a double-blind experiment or, in full, a double-blind, randomised placebo-controlled test. The results showed that more than two-thirds of the patients displayed an improvement of their symptoms, irrespective of whether they had undergone the real or the fake operation.

It is difficult to say to what extent the placebo effect contributes to the success of surgery in general. It is probably more significant than we think. Fortunately, thanks to double-blind, randomised placebo-controlled testing, operations like that performed on Alan B. Shepard, which have purely a placebo effect, are performed less and less frequently. In the past, however, the outcomes of operations were not systematically recorded and the scientific publication of surgical results was usually limited to descriptions of successful individual cases rather than presenting

Location and direction in the body

An exact anatomical indication of location and direction is
essential for good communication between doctors. To do
that, they use a whole arsenal of Latin and Greek terms. It is
these terms that make surgical jargon so incomprehensible to
the layman. Anterior and ventral (towards the *venter*, belly)
both refer to the front, posterior and dorsal (towards the *dorsum*,
back) to the back. Cranial means upwards (towards the *cranium*,
head), caudal means downwards (towards the *cauda*, tail). Lateral
means to the side, medial to the middle. The eyes are thus
lateral to the nose, medial to the ears and cranial to the mouth.
Combinations are also possible, such as anteromedial or postero-
caudal. Proximal and distal mean closer or further away from
the core of the body, respectively. So the elbow is distal from
the shoulder, but proximal to the wrist. Superior and supra-
mean above, while inferior, sub- and infra- mean below. Intra-
is in, inter- is between, para- is next to, juxta- is near to,
endo- means inside, exo- and extra- outside, retro- behind,
per- and trans- through or via, and peri- around. Central and
peripheral speak for themselves, median means on the midline.
Volar and palmar both mean on the palm side of the hand,
i.e. anterior if the thumb points laterally. The sole of the foot
is plantar. The thumb side of the hand is radial, the little finger
side is ulnar and the back of the hand is dorsal, as is the top
of the foot. The sagittal plane divides the body into left and
right halves – the plane in which an arrow strikes you (*sagitta*
is Latin for arrow). The frontal plane divides the body into
front and back and the axial or transverse plane into a top
and bottom half. In medicine, surgery and anatomy left and
right are always from the patient's point of view (else you
have to specify whether you look at the patient from the front
or from the back).

average figures for large groups of patients. Surgeons performed operations if they had seen that earlier results had been favourable,

but did not critically study the results for all other patients who had undergone the same procedure. This was the reason why, for many centuries, a pure placebo procedure – bloodletting – was the most commonly performed surgical operation.

Bloodletting was used as a cure-all for practically everything: wound infections, fever and even, counter-intuitively, severe bleeding. Although a large number of patients died not despite, but *because* of, bloodletting, it must have had a beneficial effect for some, or it would have been abandoned much earlier. However, that benefit must have been a purely placebo effect, as there is absolutely no demonstrable evidence of bloodletting being beneficial in medical terms. In other words, if Alan B. Shepard and his surgeon had believed in bloodletting, Shepard could just as easily have gone to the Moon after being bled as by undergoing the much more complex operation on his inner ear.

It was usually the job of the surgeon or barber – the men with the knives – who performed bloodletting. The tradition must have originated thousands of years ago with exorcism rituals, where medicine men would drive out evil spirits (diseases) by cutting the victim open. The ancient Greeks practised libation: a sacrifice offered by spilling red wine on the ground. Bloodletting was thus comparable to making a sacrifice. And since loss of blood could cause the victim to faint, they seemed to be in a trance or surrendering to the gods. Superstitious belief in evil spirits continued to be an important component of bloodletting until well into the Middle Ages but, in the centuries that followed, surgeons preferred a more rational explanation: it was a matter of ridding the body of blood 'corrupted' by disease or infection. One way of doing this was to place a tourniquet around the upper arm and tapping blood off through an incision in the elbow. (This is where the expression 'bad blood' comes from.)

The special knife used for bloodletting was called a fleam. It was designed so that it would not cut too deep. The favourite place to make an incision was in the fold of the elbow, because of the vein there just below the surface. Unfortunately, not much deeper than the vein, is the main artery to the arm. So, if the surgeon cut even slightly too deep, the bloodletting would turn into a bloodbath. The aponeurosis (flat tendon, or fascia) that happens to pass between these two blood vessels offers at least some protection, and was therefore also referred to as the *fascie grâce à Dieu*, the 'praise be to God' fascia.

A healthy body can replenish about one session of bloodletting a day with new blood but, after a week, the body's iron reserves will be almost depleted. In the history of medicine the fashion for bloodletting is not one to look upon with any pleasure. We can of course forgive old doctors and healers for not being able to cure diseases and heal wounds through a lack of knowledge and understanding, but intentionally inflicting fatal wounds because you don't know a better alternative is absurd. Bloodletting continued until the end of the nineteenth century, when it quietly died out, perhaps because, as more and more real treatments were found for a growing variety of diseases and ailments, doctors and surgeons no longer believed in its beneficial properties and its placebo effect became less effective.

After bloodletting had been abandoned, however, more operations were developed that we would now consider as pure placebo procedures. In the nineteenth century, at an advanced age, French physiologist Charles-Édouard Brown-Séquard injected himself with a potion concocted from the testicles of guinea pigs and announced that it had a rejuvenating effect. With such experiments, he laid the basis for endocrinology, a branch of medical science that deals with hormones, and surgeons started implanting patients with slivers of animal testicles for their rejuvenative properties, with surprisingly beneficial effects. But many more recent operations rely to a greater or lesser extent on a placebo effect, including removing the uvula to relieve sleeping problems or varicose veins in patients with restless legs, hernia operations to alleviate chronic back pain, anti-reflux surgery for people with chest pains, implanting spinal electrodes for chronic pain, operating on the blood vessels in the penis to cure impotence, laparoscopic groin hernia operations on athletes with pain in the groin, brain operations on Parkinson's patients, and operating on tennis elbow.

When operations are performed to alleviate inexplicable chronic symptoms, a beneficial result is more often due to a placebo effect than a real solution to the problem. The medical term for symptoms for which no clear cause can be found is *e causa ignota* or e.c.i., Latin for 'of unknown cause'. Chronic abdominal pains are a good example of a problem treated by a wide variety of operations, even when they are e.c.i. One suspicious fact is that these procedures seem to work best when they are new. They tend to come in fits and starts, as fashionable fads. New simply seems better than old, and innovations usually imply promises. In the 1960s and 1970s, for example, it was popular to remove healthy appendices to treat chronic abdominal pains e.c.i. In the 1980s and 1990s it was believed that these inexplicable complaints could be relieved by severing adhesions in the abdominal cavity. For exactly the same symptoms, it is nowadays fashionable to cut through superficial nerves in the abdominal wall, and no one operates any more to sever adhesions or remove a healthy appendix.

Surgeons have a tendency to attribute the observed beneficial effects of their treatment almost exclusively to their own actions. 'The patient came to me with a problem,' they might say. 'I applied a treatment that I was certain would help. The patient went home satisfied with no more symptoms. That was a good result of my work. But that was to be expected, of course.' This way of thinking and working based on overconfidence in one's own actions is known as self-serving bias. A surgeon should actually ask himself after every operation whether the patient no longer suffers from the symptoms because of the operation, or in spite of it. Perhaps the symptoms would have gone away by themselves? Perhaps the symptoms return later, but the patient does not come back to the surgeon? The only genuine way to determine the value of a treatment is to distance oneself from the one-to-one relationship between patient and surgeon.

The true value of a surgical procedure can only be determined objectively with large groups of patients all undergoing the same operation for the same problem, preferably conducted by different surgeons in different hospitals. In modern surgery, this value is then adopted in national or international guidelines based on such results. The guidelines have to be reviewed regularly, as new insights can be acquired from new results from new groups of patients.

If specific operations prove to be placebo procedures, it is not worth continuing to perform them, even though many patients benefit from them, because they are unnecessarily expensive and generate unnecessary expectations. Moreover, in many cases, they do not work at all or only temporarily, and if they do seem to work, it may be that the symptoms would have disappeared anyway. Many chronic symptoms come and go with a rhythm that cannot always be explained. And, of course, it is not a good thing to deceive patients with a treatment that is not a real treatment. Every operation – including a placebo – runs the risk of complications and it is not acceptable to use a fake procedure that happens to be in trend.

But even when procedures are exposed as placebo, it can take time for them to go out of fashion. This is the case with arthroscopy (keyhole surgery) on patients suffering from gonarthrosis (osteoarthritis of the knee), which was exposed as a placebo operation in 2002. The operation has become very popular based on patients' responses to it, though in fact very little is done to the knee, besides inspecting, rinsing and cleaning it a little.

To test this, Bruce Moseley, an orthopaedic surgeon in Houston in the United States, performed a fake arthroscopy of the knee on a large group of patients. Moseley made three small incisions in the skin and, in full view of the patient, played around with a wide range of instruments and spilled rinsing fluid on the floor to make it all look as real as possible. The results were astounding. Arthroscopic rinsing of a worn knee joint, laboriously scraping wear and tear from the cartilage and neatly smoothing a damaged meniscus proved to have just as much effect on the pain and as little effect on the functioning of the joint as pretending to do so. And yet, keyhole surgery to the knee continues to be the most commonly performed orthopaedic procedure in the world. Hobbling to a private orthopaedic clinic to have your worn-out knee looked at now seems little different from taking a good slug of Lourdes water, lighting a candle at the statue of the Virgin in 's-Hertogenbosch, or going to the barber to be bled. All you have to do is believe in it.

Twelve men have stood on the Moon – Neil Armstrong, Buzz Aldrin, Pete Conrad, Alan Bean, Alan B. Shepard, Edgar Mitchell, David Scott, James Irwin, John Young, Charles Duke, Harrison Schmitt and Eugene Cernan. Of them all, Shepard was the oldest. Imagine that, despite his endolymphatic-shunt operation, he had experienced symptoms of his disease while he was up there. He could have choked if he had vomited while wearing his helmet. After the drama of Apollo 13, that would have meant a definite end to the lunar missions. It is not known if he suffered symptoms of Ménière's disease after returning to earth. Shepard died of leukaemia in 1998.

21

Umbilical Hernia

The Miserable Death of a Stout Lady: Queen Caroline

THE ANCIENT GREEK philosophers hit the nail on the head with their ideas about how the world works. From the very beginning, they encompassed the whole of science in one simple principle: nothing is certain, everything changes, all the time. In the sixth century BC, Heraclitus expressed this idea in the phrase *panta rhei*, 'everything flows'. If you look at a river for a second time, it is still the same river, but the water is different.

Living beings, too, are flowing rivers that are continually changing, without altering their form. No one knows that better than a doctor. For a patient with symptoms that you cannot explain, there is no better cure than to wait. As most ailments will simply go away by themselves, your doctor has good reason to bide his time and ask you to come back after a few days. There is also no better way of making a diagnosis than waiting to see which way the problems 'flow'. The secret is, of course, to know when it is the right moment to stop waiting and start treating the patient.

Waiting is also a valuable instrument in surgery, both in making a diagnosis and in improving the patient's state of health. This is reflected in the three different approaches that a surgeon can adopt in treating a patient: conservative (treating without surgical intervention), expectative (watchful waiting without treating) and invasive (intervening surgically in the flow of events). Waiting is often a wise course of action if you know what you are doing, but it can be difficult to persuade the suffering patient, a concerned family, and colleagues who think they know better, why you don't seem to be doing anything. Doing nothing is, after all, not what many people expect a surgeon to do. But a well-thought-out decision to wait calls for just as much nerve as taking action, and whether a surgeon is a good doctor or not depends not on taking prompt surgical steps, but on the result. That is why a good surgeon knows the course followed by every disease and disorder, so that he does not wait too long, nor intervene too soon.

The course of a wound infection is a few days; if there is no pus by then, then no pus will develop. The course of cancer is a number of months; if there is no tumour by then, there was no tumour in the first place. The course of a leaking intestinal anastomosis (where two parts of the intestine have been joined together surgically) is ten days; if it has not leaked by then, it will not leak at all. The course of a fully blocked artery in the leg is six hours; if the leg has not died off by then, it will survive. You can safely leave an ileus (an obstruction in the small intestine) for several days before it ruptures, but if you discover a colon obstruction (a blockage in the large intestine), you have no time to sleep on it. However, a blockage in any intestine with strangulation of the bowel is life-threatening within a few hours because the intestinal wall will die from lack of blood supply.

Eighteenth-century surgeon John Ranby waited too long before treating the symptoms of Queen Caroline, wife of George II. Subsequently, he failed to observe a favourable development in the course of her illness and believed that he had to take action after all. That cost his patient her life. But, because neither he nor anyone else in the eighteenth century had any idea at all what was wrong with the queen, no one blamed him and he was even knighted because he had eventually stuck his scalpel in her navel. Better late than never, they must have thought.

Queen Caroline called him a 'blockhead'. John Ranby had been a member of the Company of Barber-Surgeons in London and, when a separate Company of Surgeons was set up in 1745, he became its first Master. This was the first association of real surgeons and would later become the prestigious Royal College of Surgeons. Ranby was an inelegant, oafish man who, despite being well respected by the upper-class elite, would mark up few successes in his surgical life.

Caroline of Brandenburg-Ansbach was of noble descent. She married George Augustus, the eldest son of George Louis, the Prince-Elector of Hanover, later George I of Great Britain. When Queen Anne died in 1714, the distant Hanoverian branch of the English royal family was the only one that still had Protestant progeny. So George senior was put on a boat to England, together with his son and daughter-in-law Caroline, to become king. On their arrival, the German family suddenly found themselves at the centre of the highly fashionable English periwig era, which was to be named the 'Georgian Age' after them.

The royal family spoke French to each other and, in public, incomprehensible English with a heavy German accent. The two Georges, both notorious pile-sufferers, were boorish, dull and moody. The princess, on the other hand, was completely the opposite. Interesting, charming, witty and very beautiful, Caroline and her ladies-in-waiting became the high point of glamour and style. The mantua was in fashion, a grotesque dress with enormous side-extensions on both hips supported by whalebone stiffeners, so wide that the ladies could not pass through an open door without turning sideways. They would also wear a very high wig on their heads, painted their necks and faces bright white with a thick layer of toxic lead pigment, completing the picture with a black beauty spot above the corner of the mouth. They would then be stuffed – wig, dress and all – into a one-person sedan chair carried by two lackeys and rushed around London from one ball to the next. When she was older, however, Caroline no longer fitted into her sedan chair, or her dress for that matter.

George I died of a stroke in the summer of 1727 in the coach to Osnabrück. He had spent all night on the toilet in the Dutch town of Delden, where he had developed indigestion after eating too many strawberries during a stop en route to Hanover. The new King George II and his consort, Queen Caroline, had waited thirteen years for the throne. In all those years of luxury and idleness, the once so beautiful Caroline had become hopelessly obese. Although her true size was never shown in portraits and the fame of her enormous breasts was ultimately greater than they were in reality, once Caroline finally became queen, she was so immense that she could no longer turn over in bed without the aid of her servants. Her husband, the king, took a mistress – his wife's head lady-in-waiting no less – but no matter how unhappy this made the queen, she continued to love him, and he her.

Caroline was probably not ashamed of her gluttony or her body. Normal citizens could buy tickets to watch the royal couple eat their meals on Sundays. People could see the queen, with her immensely obese body, gorge herself. But she carried a secret that only her husband knew about. As a result of all that excess weight and a series of pregnancies, after the birth of her youngest daughter, Princess Louise, a swelling had developed in the centre of her abdomen. She skilfully concealed this bulge beneath her clothing. It was an umbilical hernia that had eventually grown to an 'immense size'. No one knows just how large it was but, especially with people who are overweight, an umbilical hernia can be enormous, as large as a water melon, for example. Some can become so big that, sagging under their own weight, they hang down to the knees like an elongated sac.

Acid

A large number of systems in our bodies necessarily have to be able to work together for us to survive. Our metabolism, respiration, blood coagulation, immunological resistance, digestion, the production of body fluids and hormones by the glands, the absorption of nutrients, the elimination of toxic waste, the circulatory system of the blood, the working of the muscles, thinking, cell division and tissue growth, water management, the distribution of minerals, and a whole range of other functions all need each other to continue to work properly. For that to happen, our bodies must create a constant environment in which all these systems can operate optimally. Our body temperature has to be maintained at 37°C and the ideal acidity level of the body (pH) is 7.4 (a little less acid than pure water). Our metabolism and respiration produce acidic waste by burning calories, including lactic acid and carbon dioxide (CO_2). Excess acid is removed from the blood by the kidneys and through exhalation. Toxins produced by dead tissue and bacteria are also acidic. A patient suffering from a serious infection or whose cells are dying off will start to breathe more rapidly to compensate for the excess of acid being produced by expelling (exhaling) more carbon dioxide. If the patient is too exhausted to expel any more CO_2, the level of acid in the blood will rise to a critical level. This is known as acidosis. It has an immediate detrimental effect on all of the body's systems. As these systems fail, the pH level in the body will fall even further – a downward spiral that ends in death.

An umbilical hernia occurs when the intestines or internal organs protrude (or herniate) from the abdominal cavity through the navel (umbilicus) in the muscles of the abdominal wall. The navel opening is left after birth and is normally less than half a centimetre in diameter, small enough to withstand the pressure in the abdomen. If, however, the contents of the abdomen expand for a long period, for example due to excess fatty tissue or multiple pregnancies, the umbilical opening can weaken and stretch. Consequently the abdominal content can be pushed through the enlarged opening; over time, more and more abdominal content can be pushed out.

If the umbilical opening continues to widen, the protruding intestines retain sufficient space in the hernia not to be constricted. The bulge is then merely inconvenient and only painful when pressure in the abdomen suddenly rises, for example during coughing, sneezing, laughing or straining. When the patient lies on her back, gravity will decrease the pressure in the hernia so that the intestines can fall back to their original position in the abdomen and the swelling will disappear until the patient stands up again. This is known as spontaneous reduction. But even a spontaneously reducing umbilical hernia will never go away of its own accord. Sooner or later, more abdominal tissue will find its way into the hernia. The symptoms will then worsen and the swelling will no longer disappear when the patient lies on their back. The hernia is then no longer reducible. If more abdominal content is forced into the hernia, it can become constricted. That will cause sudden severe pain and vomiting. Also the tissue in the hernia will die if nothing is done to reduce the pressure in the umbilical opening. The hernia is then incarcerated, from the Latin *incarcerare* meaning 'to imprison', and its contents are strangulated. The outcome of an incarcerated hernia depends on what kind of tissue is strangulated, the surgeon who addresses the problem and, especially, at what point he does that.

In the summer of 1737, Caroline had severe pain in the abdomen twice, but both times it passed away on its own. On the morning of Wednesday 9 November, she again experienced extreme pain, which would persist until she died, eleven days later. What happened in and around the queen's bedroom in those days was recorded in great detail in the memoirs of Lord John Hervey, Vice Chamberlain and a personal friend of the royal couple. The queen's pain was acute and unbearable, and was accompanied by vomiting. And yet she insisted on appearing in the drawing room that evening as usual. During the night, she continued to retch, could not lie still, and the mint water and herbal bitters administered to her did not stay down. Royal surgeon John Ranby was summoned, and he took austere measures: he gave Caroline usquebaugh (whisky) to drink and immediately bled her twelve ounces.

The following day was a busy one for Ranby. He started by letting more blood from the queen, as she was still not feeling any better. Then he had to attend to Caroline's daughter Caroline, who had spent so long sobbing at her mother's bedside that she had a nosebleed. Ranby was in no doubt about how to treat the distressed young lady. He bled her, too – twice for good measure. Meanwhile, the queen was plagued by all kinds of doctors administering all kinds of treatments. They raised blisters on her legs, made her drink elixirs and rinsed her bowel, despite the fact that no one knew what was wrong with her. They attributed it all to 'gout of the stomach'. One of the doctors was slapped by the king for suggesting that the queen might not recover.

On the Friday morning, the queen was bled again, but the pain continued and she vomited everything she tried to eat or drink. On the Saturday, the king could no longer keep up the pretence and revealed his wife's secret. Much against her will, he told Ranby about the umbilical hernia that she had concealed for more than thirteen years. Only then – the fourth day of her illness – was the patient examined. Ranby felt the swelling on her abdomen and immediately summoned two fellow surgeons, a court surgeon called Busier, who was nearly ninety, and the much younger John Shipton, surgeon of the city. While the three physicians tended to the queen, George II started to organise his wife's estate. The situation was finally being taken seriously.

Busier suggested an extensive operation, cutting the umbilical opening deep down in the hernia so that the strangulated bowels could be pushed back into the abdomen. This showed that the aged surgeon still possessed a sharp surgical mind, but he was clearly way ahead of his time, as Ranby opposed the suggestion and Shipton agreed with the latter's advice to wait a little longer. The patient's pain increased as the day wore on, however, and in the early evening Ranby proposed the incomprehensible compromise of making an incision, but no deeper than the skin. Around six o'clock, the three eighteenth-century specialists performed the operation by candlelight, standing around the bed of the brave queen. She was accustomed to sleeping on five mattresses. This must have made the operation very taxing on the backs of the three surgeons, who not only had to bend over the pile of mattresses but also over the enormous bulk of their patient. Ranby's jacket was soaked with sweat. Like three medical students letting themselves go on a corpse in the dissecting room, they cut open the skin of the bulging umbilicus and tried to push the now visible contents back into the queen's abdomen. These must have been the most painful moments in the queen's life, but their efforts were in vain. The result was even more miserable: the most prominent woman in the country now not only had a strangulated umbilical hernia but also a large, gaping wound.

Although the three surgeons were concerned – and with very good reason – about how this horrific situation would ultimately end, they overlooked the clear sign of the favourable course of the queen's illness. If the bowel really had been incarcerated, Caroline would never have survived those five long days. The dead intestinal wall would have allowed the toxic waste of the mortified cells, the digestive fluids and the contents of the intestines into the blood within a few hours. That would have caused a disastrous biochemical chain reaction during which the increased acidity would cause havoc in all of the systems in her body in no time. She would certainly have died within two days at the most. But on Sunday 13 November, she was still very much alive, awake and responding to those around her bed. There must therefore have been something else trapped in her umbilical opening.

Especially in cases of obesity, there is a large structure hanging in front of the intestines in the abdominal cavity, known as the greater omentum or epiploon. That is normally a thin membrane between the abdominal wall and the bowels, but in severely obese people enormous quantities of fatty tissue accumulate in it. What was trapped in the queen's umbilical hernia was therefore more likely to be her greater omentum than her intestines. The difference is that, though a strangulated omentum is painful, it is less dangerous because the mortified fat cells make the victim less sick than a dead, rotting bowel.

On Sunday, the day after the operation, the surgeons tended to the painful wound. Because they could now see better in daylight than in the candlelight of the previous evening, they suddenly noticed the mortified fat tissue deep in the hernia. In those days, any mortification in a wound was normally taken to be a sure sign that the patient would die a quick death from gangrene. So, although the queen felt no worse than the day before and there were no other signs of her imminent demise, the three surgeons believed that she now had no longer than a few hours to live. The king was called to take his leave of her. He was inconsolable. He promised to always stay faithful to his beloved wife, even after her death, despite her exhortations to marry again. Sobbing and snivelling, George II uttered the historic words '*Non, j'aurai des maîtresses*' ('No, I shall have mistresses), to which Caroline replied, sighing, '*Ah! Mon Dieu! Cela n'empêche pas*' ('My God, that won't make any difference!').

The surgeons returned to their work. As they cut away dead tissue, they again failed to notice the favourable sign that no faeces came out of the wound, meaning that what they were cutting away was not intestine. Vice Chamberlain Lord Hervey became increasingly agitated by the shameless indifference with which the surgeons dealt with the emotions of the patient and her loved ones. Only a few hours previously, they had announced that the queen was nearing her end, and now that had not happened the three men were acting as though nothing was wrong. The mortifying tissue in her umbilical hernia had little immediate effect on the queen and, in the days that followed, she received both the prime minister and the archbishop. She was, however, becoming weaker. She could still not keep any food down and had to vomit constantly. The surgeons operated on her every day, tended to the wound, cut away dead tissue, sticking their fingers in it and fathoming it with probes, all of course without any form of anaesthetic. During one of these procedures, the aged Busier had held the candle a little too close to his head and his wig had caught fire. The newspapers published every horrific detail and Caroline's case was publicly debated, in Hervey's words, 'as if she had been dissected before [the palace] gate'.

The situation did not really take a turn for the worse until Thursday 17 November when the bowels must have punctured. The vomiting increased and a large quantity of faeces suddenly started flowing out of the wound. As the ordure gushed out of the queen's belly, soaking her sheets and pouring over the floor of her bedroom, the windows were thrown open because of the stench. And yet she lasted another three long days, dying at ten o'clock in the evening on Sunday 20 November 1737 in the filthiest and most miserable of circumstances. She was fifty-four years old.

How would the queen's symptoms have been explained with our present-day knowledge? The most important clue is the abnormal course of her illness. From the beginning, she suffered from an ileus, a blockage in the small intestine. That is compatible with strangulation of the intestine in an incarcerated umbilical hernia. But, as the hole in the intestine only occurred after eight days, it could not have been caused by strangulation, because that would have led to disaster after only a few hours. Perhaps the ileus had gone on for too long, the pressure had risen too high and the small intestine had burst like a balloon. It is, however, more likely to have been caused by the three surgeons rummaging around in the depths of the queen's abdomen. During their daily operations, they could have easily made a hole in the bowel, which was already under pressure. The fact that the queen was constantly vomiting strongly suggests a blockage of the intestine. Her small intestine was thus pinched together, perhaps by being trapped in the umbilical opening together with the greater omentum, but without being strangulated. The blockage could also have originated deeper in the abdomen, if the omentum had been pulling on the intestine.

In any case, at a time when surgeons often did more harm than good, the only correct treatment would have been to push the hernia back into the abdomen without operating. Ranby should not have waited to do that, but have insisted from the first day on examining the sick woman and not bleeding her without first assessing the situation. He should then have exerted gentle pressure on the swelling with flat hands for at least half an hour to try to push the umbilical bulge, at least partially, back into the abdomen. He did not even have to do that to save the mortifying content of the hernia, as that was clearly not threatening the queen's life, but only to relieve the obstruction in the small intestine. Once he had cut into it, however, all hope was lost.

Fourteen years later, on 19 December 1751, history repeated itself in Denmark. Princess Louise, one of Caroline's daughters, married the Danish king and became a queen. Like her mother, Louise was obese. At the age of twenty-seven, while pregnant, she too developed an incarcerated umbilical hernia. And again a surgeon made a futile attempt to save her. In the same gruesome circumstances as her mother, she lost both her young life and her child.

Despite this debacle at the beginning of his career, John Ranby had a very high opinion of himself. He described his most glorious moments as a sergeant-surgeon in the English army in the years that followed in his book *The Method of Treating Gunshot Wounds*, published in 1744. One of his heroic deeds was the treatment of Prince William, the youngest son of King George II and the late Queen Caroline, also known as 'The Butcher'. William fought alongside his father against the French at the Battle of Dettingen in 1743, during the War of the Austrian Succession. It was the last time in English history that the king personally led his troops on the battlefield. William was hit by a musket ball that went right through his calf, creating a wound 'as large as a chicken's egg'. Ranby immediately rushed to help the prince, who was bleeding profusely, and drew his knife. Today, a sensible surgeon would cut open the soldier's trouser leg to assess the wound, use the trouser leg to make a robust pressure bandage to stem the flow of blood, and remove the victim from the tumult of the battle as quickly as possible. But Ranby used his knife for something else. He made an incision in the fallen prince's arm to bleed him, there, in the middle of the battlefield, with musket balls flying around their ears. He drained more than half a litre of blood, as though the victim was not already losing enough blood from his leg. In the field hospital, he tended to the wound with a dressing of bread and milk and bled the prince twice more for good measure. Despite all this, the young man survived, much to the honour and relief of the surgeon. Later on Ranby would be less fortunate with his absurd style of treatment. He had caused Robert

Walpole, the British prime minister, to bleed while trying to remove a bladder stone through the urethra. Here, too, he could think of nothing better than to draw more blood from the patient, who was already bleeding to death.

22

Short Stay, Fast Track

Rebels and Revolutions: Bassini and Lichtenstein

MEDICINE, ANATOMY AND surgery make abundant use of eponyms, names derived from the person who first invented or described an instrument, anatomical structure, condition, illness or operational procedure. Italian eponyms are indisputably the most enchanting: the Finochietto retractor, the Mingazzini test, the Donati stitch, the Scopinaro procedure, the Monteggia fracture, the sphincter of Oddi, the lacunae of Morgagni, Pacchioni's granulations, the fascia of Scarpa, the Valsalva manoeuvre and the Bassini repair. It was in Italy – Padua, to be more precise – that genuine insight into how the human body functioned first developed. There, in the sixteenth century, a man from Brussels called Andries van Wezel broke the thousand-year-old tradition of uncritically applying ancient wisdom from books. He started cutting into corpses to find out the truth for himself. In his renowned book *De Humani Corporis Fabrica* (*On the Fabric of the Human Body*), published in 1543, Van Wezel – better known by his Latinised name Andreas Vesalius – showed not only how the human body is constructed but also that, for more than a thousand years, the wisdom in all the old books had been completely wrong.

Two hundred years later, at the same university in the same city, Giovanni Battista Morgagni did the same thing again, but now focusing on the diseased human body. He was the first to describe the course of diseases in living patients, and then to conduct autopsies after the patients died to see what had been wrong with them. Like that of Vesalius, his 1761 book *De Sedibus et causis morborum per anatomem indagatis* (*Of the Seats and Causes of Diseases Investigated through Anatomy*) was a great success. It was thanks to the work of these two men that medical science could develop based on facts, rather than on tradition.

But then the focus of scientific development shifted to other countries. Italy came under the influence of large foreign powers that intervened in its domestic politics and enjoyed fighting out their wars on the Italian peninsula. The country of Italy as we know it today has only been in existence since 1870. Before that, it was a collection of individual kingdoms and republics. The south was part of the French empire. In the middle was the Papal State, under the rule of the pope. The north was divided into a number of small states under the influence of yet other states. The unification of all these separate parts was partly due to the efforts of bandit and guerrilla fighter Giuseppe Garibaldi. Garibaldi led a small army of nationalists, who fought against both the French and the pope. France soon retreated, needing its armies more urgently in its war against Germany, but the pope succeeded in delaying the inevitable for another three years with a victory over a small group of freedom fighters in Rome in 1867.

In 1861, Pope Pius IX had called on all Catholics around the world to come and fight for the Papal State. Those who heeded the call were assigned to an army unit known as the Papal Zouaves. It was one of the Papal Zouaves who wounded a soldier from Garibaldi's small army in the right groin with his bayonet. That unfortunate freedom fighter was Edoardo Bassini, a twenty-one-year-old recently graduated doctor who had joined the nationalists as an infantryman. His uncle had fought shoulder-to-shoulder with Garibaldi and had become a national hero. Under the leadership of the valiant Cairoli brothers, Edoardo and his unit of seventy men had advanced within reach of Rome. They could see the dome of St Peter's Basilica on the horizon. With 300 men, the Zouaves were in the majority when the opposing parties met in the orchards of Villa Glori, on a hill a few kilometres from the Tiber in the late afternoon of 23 October 1867. The skirmish – which lasted about an hour – became known as the 'scontro di Villa Glori' (clash of Villa Glori) and led to a temporary suspension of the campaign against the Papal State.

So there he lay, the young Edoardo Bassini, under an almond tree near Rome in the autumn sun, with a gaping wound in his groin. Perhaps the doctor investigated the severity of his injury with his finger. It was not bleeding heavily, but the hole was deep, passing right through his abdominal muscles. It must have given him a particularly good view of the various layers of his abdominal wall and he would have been able to feel each of them individually. It may have been there, under that tree, that the idea was born that would later make him so famous.

Bassini was taken as a prisoner-of-war and treated, under guard, by former professor of surgery Luigi Porta in the university hospital in Pavia. The wound was down in the right lower abdomen and started to leak faeces. Bassini developed life-threatening peritonitis, but after a few days his fever retreated and the flow of excrement from the wound lessened. The bayonet had apparently pierced his caecum, the short cul de sac of intestine at the beginning of the great bowel. If it had been a little lower, the large blood vessels to his leg would have been pierced and he would have bled to death under the almond tree. A little higher and the large intestine would have been damaged and Edoardo would not have survived the peritonitis. He was extremely lucky – he recovered fully from his injuries and was set free a few months later.

Having lost his taste for fighting, Bassini rediscovered his interest in surgery and set out to learn more. He went to see all the great surgeons of his time: Theodor Billroth in Vienna, Bernhard von Langenbeck in Berlin and Joseph Lister in London. Back in the now-unified Italy, he became a professor at the University of Padua, the city of Morgagni and Vesalius. There, in 1887, he presented his fundamental solution to a problem that had not been solved in more than 3,000 years of surgery: how to treat a groin hernia.

A groin hernia is one of the most common conditions affecting humans. The mummy of Pharaoh Rameses V, who died in 1157 BC, shows clear signs of a groin hernia. The medical term is inguinal hernia, literally meaning 'a breach of the groin'. Twenty-five per cent of men and three per cent of women will develop a groin hernia at some point in their lives. The cause is a congenital weak spot in the left and right lower abdominal wall.

The abdominal wall comprises three muscles lying one on top of the other. That is clear to see in the different layers in a slice of bacon. From the inside to the outside, these are the transverse abdominal muscle, the internal oblique muscle and the external oblique muscle. On both sides of the body, there is a hole in each of these three layers of muscle. Together, these three holes form a tunnel known as the inguinal canal.

Men are more likely to contract a hernia than women because, before they are born, their testicles have passed through the inguinal canal on their way from the abdomen to the scrotum. That can weaken its resistance to the high pressure in the abdominal cavity. In some cases, the inguinal canal is already so weak at birth that a groin hernia can develop in the early years of life. It can, however, still be robust enough to withstand the pressure for many years and only rupture much later. That is why groin hernias are most common among young children and the elderly.

That weak spot where the intestines protrude is known as the hernial gate. A hernia of the groin is also known as a rupture, but that term is misleading. A rupture of the abdominal wall refers only to the inguinal gate, and that in itself is not the problem. A groin hernia only causes complaints or complications

Hernia

Hernia is Latin for rupture. Although the word rupture suggests a tear or a crack, the medical term for these is not hernia, but fissure. Hernia is used only for a tear or crack through which something protrudes. It is used for two completely different conditions. A crack can develop in one of the intervertebral discs in the spine, through which the soft core of the disc (the nucleus pulposus) can protrude. This is known as a *hernia nuclei pulposi*, spinal disc herniation or a 'slipped disc'. If the protrusion presses against one of the nerve roots that leave the spine from the spinal cord, it can cause a radiating pain in the area supplied by that nerve root. In the case of a back hernia, the pain therefore radiates to the leg while, with a neck hernia, it radiates to the arm. The second form of hernia is the protrusion of the peritoneum through a rupture or weak spot in the abdominal wall. With an umbilical hernia, this weak spot is the umbilical opening, through which the umbilical cord once passed. In the case of a diaphragmatic hernia, it is the hole where the oesophagus passes through the diaphragm. With an incisional hernia, the weak spot is an old scar while, with a femoral hernia, it is the hole through which the blood vessels pass from the abdomen to the leg. With a groin hernia, the weak spot is the inguinal canal, through which – in the case of men – the testicles have moved down to the scrotum. That is why groin hernias are more common among men.

if the contents of the abdominal cavity start herniating through the ruptured wall. The protruding intestines are still surrounded by the peritoneum. This is called the hernial sac. The protrusion of the hernial sac through the hernial gate (the inguinal canal) can be seen or felt on the outside as a subcutaneous swelling just above the groin crease. When the patient lies flat on his back, the hernial sac and intestines fall back inside and the swelling disappears. As with an umbilical hernia, the intestines can also become trapped in the hernial gate and strangulated. That causes a life-threatening incarcerated groin hernia.

Until Bassini, the treatment of a groin hernia focused on the result of the hernia rather than its cause; in other words, on the protruding hernial sac, but not on the hernial gate. The Mesopotamians, Egyptians and Greeks already had trusses to press groin hernias back inside and, from Roman times until well after the Middle Ages, groin hernias were also treated surgically. Firstly, the swelling could be seared from the outside with a branding iron. The benefit of this almost inhuman treatment is, however, not clear. It was probably applied simply because that was what was prescribed in the thousand-year-old book by the Arab surgeon Albucasis. Secondly, there was the real operation, which was already performed before the start of the Common Era. That entailed making an incision over the swelling, holding the hernial sac at the top, twisting it and stitching it up to seal it off. In the fourteenth century, French surgeon Guy de Chauliac preferred to use a golden thread for this procedure. The testicle would often die off following the operation. In the case of an incarcerated groin hernia, the patient was hung upside down to make the incision in the swelling, so that the contents of the hernia could be pushed back inside more easily. If, however, the incarcerated intestine was already strangulated, the patient would usually die. In the nineteenth century, methods improved as surgeons started working more hygienically and patients were anaesthetised. Nevertheless, until Bassini, they would still restrict themselves to removing the hernial sac, without treating the hernial gate. Consequently, there was always a risk that the problem would recur within a short time.

Bassini realised that the hernial sac was not the cause of the problem, but the effect. He focused on the cause, the weak spot, and spent many years studying the different layers of the inguinal canal. The basis of the Bassini procedure was restoration of the original anatomy of the abdominal wall after removing the hernial sac. This idea of operating not only to fix what was wrong but also restore the normal situation was new in surgery.

To reconstruct the original situation, however, you need to know exactly what that situation was. That means not only knowing what the body looks like normally (i.e. the normal anatomy of the abdominal wall), but how it has been changed by the groin hernia. It was therefore a happy coincidence that Bassini worked out his idea in Padua, at the university where Vesalius had laid out the basis for normal, and Morgagni for abnormal, anatomy. Bassini described his method in 1889 as a '*nuovo metodo operativo per la cura radicale dell'ernia inguinale*', a new surgical method for the definitive repair of a groin hernia.

This was his revolutionary idea: cut open all parts that no longer comply with the normal anatomical situation and stitch them up again to reconstruct the abdominal wall as it ought to be. As he lay under the almond tree, Bassini must have been able to feel in the war wound that had gone through every layer of his own abdominal wall that this is easier said than done. He must have already understood back then that each of those layers play their own role in maintaining the solidity of the whole and therefore have to be repaired in their own way to treat a groin hernia.

Although seven different layers can be distinguished in the abdominal wall, Bassini discovered that they can be divided into three functional units, all of which have a distinct role to play in the abdominal wall and therefore have to be addressed differently in treating a groin hernia. Firstly, there is the protective covering, consisting of the skin, the subcutaneous tissue and the external oblique abdominal muscle. This layer does not contribute to the solidity of the abdominal wall, as it cannot sufficiently resist the pressure from inside the abdomen. Secondly, below the protective covering, is the muscle layer, comprising the internal oblique abdominal muscle, the transverse muscle and the transverse fascia or 'second peritoneum'. This muscular layer has to withstand the pressure in the abdomen all on its own, and is therefore the key to the problem. Below that, lastly, is the hernial sac, formed from the peritoneum. Like the first layer, the hernial sac does not contribute to the strength of the abdominal wall.

With a groin hernia, the hernial sac protrudes through the muscle layer to form a swelling which is covered only by the protective layer. Bassini first cut open all the layers of the disrupted abdominal wall (the protective layer and the muscles) and then stitched up the muscle layer with strong silk thread – just like a fat man, whose belly has burst through the buttons of his shirt and sticks out under his pullover, tries to push it back by buttoning his shirt back up and tucking it into his trousers. Bassini described 262 patients operated on with excellent results.

Unfortunately, the Bassini repair was not adequate for treating severe hernias. In many cases, the essential muscle layer is so weakened by the groin hernia that it can no longer be used for reconstruction (in other words, the shirt is too small). Then additional solidity has to be provided. Metal wire, rubber and nylon were all used, but the body could not tolerate these materials and they broke easily. The solution eventually presented itself through space travel, where materials have to comply with very high requirements. The parachutes used to brake manned spacecraft were made of a polyethylene plastic that could withstand extreme forces. This material would have been assigned to the annals of history if it had not been applied in two very prominent products.

In 1957, it was used to make hula hoops, and in 1958 surgeon Francis Usher used a woven mesh of the material to repair a groin hernia. Scar tissue fuses the synthetic material with the surrounding tissues, restoring their original solidity. Usher placed the mesh deep in the abdominal wall, between the hernial sac and the muscle layer – as though the fat man gives up on the buttons on his shirt and puts on a robust undershirt instead.

Bassini had given surgery a second objective. An operation must now not only solve a problem but also, as far as possible, restore the original situation. The next major step in treating groin hernias would again affect surgery as a whole. It was taken by Irving Lichtenstein, an American surgeon with a private clinic, the Lichtenstein Hernia Institute, on Sunset Boulevard in Beverly Hills, Los Angeles. He operated on his groin hernia patients using a variation on the regular Bassini method, but what made his procedure so exceptional was that his patients were anaesthetised locally and, after the final stitch, could get up from the operating table themselves and go straight home. That was a truly revolutionary concept. When he presented his treatment procedure in 1964, surgeons were dumbstruck. Until then, patients would spend several days, or even weeks, in a hospital bed after undergoing a groin hernia repair.

What Lichtenstein did was, figuratively speaking, exactly in line with Bassini's idea: to restore the normal situation as quickly as possible after the problem had been solved. Bassini was talking about the normal situation of the abdominal wall, Lichtenstein of the patient as a whole. That means not lying in a hospital and simply waiting, but being back at home and going about your daily business: walking, eating, drinking, taking a shower, working and so on. There proved to be no reason at all to lie in bed after a groin hernia operation.

We now know that you can not only walk around after many operations, but that it actually leads to fewer complications. In 2004, surgeons around the world were once again amazed when Danish surgeon Henrik Kehlet showed that this principle applied with major intestinal operations. Enhanced recovery, which Kehlet called 'fast-track surgery', was a combination of getting out of bed and eating and drinking normally as soon as possible, good painkillers, and 'short stay' – going home after one or two days in hospital. Until 2004, we surgeons literally forbade patients who had undergone bowel surgery to eat a single mouthful until they had passed wind. We had rinsed their intestines completely, intravenously administered fluids so that they did not have to drink and fitted a urinary catheter so that they could stay in bed and not have to get up to use the toilet. They would stay in hospital for at least two weeks, and no one was surprised when they developed strange complications like bowels that suddenly stopped working, lungs filling with fluid, bedsores and pressure ulcers or thrombosis in the legs. Since 2004, the intestines are no longer rinsed, patients are given a sandwich a couple of hours after the operation, we administer only the minimum of fluid through a drip, so that they can feel thirsty themselves and want to drink, and they get out of bed as soon as possible, for example to use the toilet without the need of a catheter. The fast-track concept has now been adopted in all branches of surgery, from groin hernia repairs to hip replacements.

The treatment for groin hernias thus advanced step by step. There would be one final step. Bassini had been wounded by a bayonet passing right through all the muscles of his abdominal wall. Although the healing of such a gaping wound must have been extremely painful, it was clear to young Bassini that you would also have to cut through all of those layers to perform a groin hernia operation. How else would you get at it? That was, of course, a serious disadvantage not only to the original Bassini procedure but also to later methods using a mesh: there was always the risk of the operation wound causing chronic pain, just as if you had been pierced with a bayonet. About a century after Bassini, that problem was also solved.

All you have to do is make sure that the mesh is fitted in the right place between the layers of the abdominal wall: above the peritoneum and below the muscle layer. It makes no difference to the outcome whether you do that via a large wound from the front or by making a detour. Thanks to laparoscopy, it is now possible to reach that point with keyhole surgery through the navel, reinforcing the abdominal wall with a mesh from the inside, without having to cut through all those seven layers. Keyhole surgery cannot, however, be conducted using local anaesthesia. But that does not have to be a disadvantage any more, thanks to the fast-track concept. After general anaesthesia, the patient can just as easily go home the same day. Groin hernia repair is currently the most frequently performed surgical procedure – and a laparoscopic operation with a mesh and a fast-track recovery is the best way to do it.

23

Mors in tabula

The Limits of Surgery: Lee Harvey Oswald

D R MALCOLM PERRY was still on duty. He was the young surgeon in Dallas who, two days previously, had experienced the most terrible moment of his short career. He had fought to save the life of President John F. Kennedy, but the horrific wounds caused by the assassin's bullets gave Perry not even the slimmest chance of success. Kennedy had died in his hands and the whole country had descended upon him.

He had not withdrawn from the limelight, not taken leave or switched shifts with his colleagues. He had just carried on working. So he was still the duty surgeon when two days later, on Sunday 24 November 1963, that strange little man – the alleged assassin himself – was brought into the same emergency room. He had just been shot and was unconscious when he arrived by ambulance. Witnesses said that he had been hit by one bullet. A breathing tube was inserted into the man's windpipe through the mouth, and he was administered blood and fluid.

There was one bullet wound visible, on the lower left side of the chest. A thorax drain was placed in his chest, a tube alongside the left lung, but no blood came out. The patient was thin and, on the opposing side of his chest, at the back and to the right, a bullet could easily be felt just below the skin. It had passed right through the upper abdomen. He still had a weak, rapid pulse of 130 beats per minute, but there was no measurable blood pressure. The man was quickly moved to the operating room, where three surgeons would fight to save his life.

The whole of America had been sitting in front of the television. They watched as the coffin of the late John F. Kennedy was driven to the Capitol in Washington, where he was to lie in state so that they could say farewell to their president. The scene switched to a garage under the police station in Dallas, where the suspected assassin was being taken to a prison van. The viewers saw a thin young man, handcuffed and led by two policemen in large cowboy hats. Suddenly, a man emerged from the throng of reporters. He approached the thin man, shoved a pistol into his ribs and shot him. It was the first murder in history to be seen live on television. The gun had been aimed at the man's heart, but he had warded off the shot and it had caught him lower in the body. With so many reporters on the spot with television and photographic cameras, the shot was recorded from several angles. Some of them can be seen on YouTube.

The gunman, Jack Ruby, was immediately overpowered by the reporters and taken to the cell that the young man had recently vacated. Amid the uproar in the garage below the police station, the cameras continued to roll. A few minutes later, an ambulance drove in and the man, clearly unconscious, was put in the back on a stretcher. There were cheers among the crowd in front of the Capitol in Washington when they heard the news of the shooting in Dallas on their transistor radios. Lee Harvey Oswald had been shot.

Oswald was taken to trauma room 2 at the Parkland Memorial Hospital in Dallas. Everyone knew the thin man's face and Malcolm Perry must have thought: 'Here we go again.'

There is a difference between elective and urgent surgery. Elective operations can be planned and do not necessarily have to be performed. In the case of urgent operations the patient has his back against the wall; it is a matter of life and death. That difference is even a little subtler: with an urgent operation, no matter how great the immediate risk of operating, it is always smaller than that of doing nothing. With an elective operation, the immediate risk of operating is always greater than doing nothing, but that gap must be acceptably small to justify operating anyway. In modern surgery, it is considered an acceptable risk if an elective operation causes complications in no more than 10 per cent of cases and the risk of death is no more than 1 per cent. Complications obviously vary widely depending on the severity of the operation, but generally serious complications occur more often with severe operations. Of course, serious complications can occur with less severe operations, but not as frequently.

The occurrence of complications after an operation is known as 'morbidity' and is expressed in percentages. General complications include wound infections, haemorrhaging, bladder or lung infections, thrombosis of the legs, a heart attack, bedsores, vomiting, constipation or an inactive small intestine. The risk of death, also expressed in percentages, is called 'mortality'. You don't die simply because of an operation or a complication. Complications are only life-threatening if they get out of hand – if they are not treated in time, or if one complication leads to another, causing a chain reaction.

Complications, even lethal complications, are a calculated risk in all operations. The patient must of course be informed of these risks in advance. Surgeon and patient reach agreement about the surgical procedures to be followed, based on the principle of informed consent. The surgeon must inform the patient about the four aspects of the operation, the patient must understand them, and they both have to agree on them. These aspects are the indication (the reason for the operation), the nature and consequences of the operation, alternatives for the operation, and all possible complications of the operation.

A complication is certainly not the same as an error. It can only be considered a surgical error if it can be attributed to incorrect action by the surgeon. If an operation is conducted *lege artis*, literally 'according to the rules of the art' (in other words, as it should be) and a problem occurs nevertheless, that is called a complication and is not an error. A complication is also different from a side effect. The first is unintentional, while the second can be expected. Side effects of an operation include pain, a high temperature, nausea, tiredness or psychological stress.

Complications in surgery relate to the skill of the surgeon, the severity of the operation, the surgical method used, the care of the patient before, during and after the operation, simple coincidence and bad luck and, last but not least, the patient himself. Not every patient is the same and the differences between them are very important in the development of complications. Complications occur more frequently with patients who are obese, who smoke, are malnourished, or have a higher biological age (not their calendar age), and where there are serious co-morbidities, that is high-risk diseases like diabetes, high blood pressure or asthma. Patients themselves can therefore reduce the risk to a certain extent themselves by, for example, giving up smoking, reducing their weight to healthy level, eating sufficient protein before the operation, and getting other diseases treated as far as possible beforehand.

Surgeons are expected to keep their own record of complications. A good complication record is a form of quality control. And yet, you cannot simply compare the results of different hospitals and surgeons. After all, a surgeon who mainly operates on cardiac patients who are old, overweight smokers is more likely to encounter complications than one whose patients are usually young and healthy.

It is a myth that surgical complications primarily occur during an operation (intra-operative). They mostly arise after the operation (post-operative). It is during an operation that a surgeon has most control over his patient and thus over a good outcome. At that moment, he holds the risks almost literally in his own hands. Because complications mostly occur later, a surgeon has to operate wearing four-dimensional glasses – the fourth dimension being time. He must be able to imagine what he now sees, dissects, reconstructs and stitches up will look like an hour, a day or a week later. If an organ, for example, is now just about receiving sufficient blood, it is not only a healthy pink colour now, but still will be in an hour's or a week's time. But if it is a little too pale, the surgeon must be able to predict whether, after a few hours, it will be black and mortified. And loss of blood can seem minimal during an operation but if it does not stop completely can accumulate over a few hours to a life-threatening level. When stitching up a hole in the intestines, the surgeon's prediction needs to be even more accurate. A repaired intestine immediately provides a watertight seal. But if the tissues of the intestinal wall around the stitching do not receive sufficient blood to heal, cells will die off in the hours or days after the operation and the intestine will leak after all.

So a surgeon has much more control during an operation than afterwards. Therefore something must go terribly wrong for a patient to die on the operating table. That is a surgeon's worst nightmare, *mors in tabula*, 'death on the table'.

The record of the surgery on Lee Harvey Oswald is a public document. It is part of the report by the Warren Commission, published in 1964, and can be found in Appendix 8 'Medical Reports from Doctors at Parkland Memorial Hospital, Dallas, Texas', as 'Commission exhibit number 392', under 'Parkland Memorial Hospital Operative Record – Lee Harvey Oswald Surgery'. The operation was performed by surgeons Tom Shires, Malcolm Perry and Robert McClelland, and chief resident Ron Jones.

They performed a xipho-pubic laparotomy, which entails opening the abdomen with the largest possible incision, along the mid-line from the point of the sternum (the xiphoid process) to the pubic bone (pubis). On opening the abdominal cavity, they immediately removed three litres of blood, including fresh clots. As the patient was in danger of bleeding to death, time was of the essence. Most of the blood seemed to be coming from the right side of the body.

In the upper right abdomen, there are five important structures in front of each other. First, the large intestine makes a bend in front of the liver, known as the hepatic flexure (literally 'liver bend'). Carefully, but as quickly as possible, they dissected that free, so that the liver was visible, with the duodenum beneath it. The large intestine and the duodenum seemed to be intact, while the liver was slightly damaged. To investigate further, the liver had to be moved aside and the duodenum dissected free. Behind that was the right kidney, which appeared at first to be seriously damaged, bleeding severely from the top. But when the surgeons dissected the kidney free to examine it more closely, they saw that most of the blood was coming from a large structure even deeper in the abdomen, the inferior vena cava, literally the 'lower hollow vein'. That is a blood vessel as thick as a thumb, with a very thin wall and directly linked to the right atrium of the heart. As all the body's blood passes through the right atrium, a hole in this major vein means that the circulatory system can literally run dry. The surgeons quickly placed a curved clamp on the blood vessel to close the hole and packed the upper right abdomen between the back, the liver and the kidney with gauzes to stem the bleeding temporarily.

It was clear to the surgeons that this was not the end of the story. There was an enormous haematoma (a localised collection of blood) in the retroperitoneum, the tissues behind the abdominal cavity. The swelling in the back of the abdomen was so extensive that the intestines were pushed out. The surgeons wanted to find out what was wrong there and decided to approach the area from the left.

In the upper left abdomen, the structures are also located in front of each other. First, the large intestine makes a bend in front of the spleen (the splenic flexure). Carefully, but as quickly as possible, the surgeons dissected this free. The spleen was then visible next to the stomach. They could see damage to the top of the spleen and, near to that, they saw a hole in the diaphragm. They dissected the stomach free and moved it aside, in order to see the pancreas, which appeared to be severely damaged. Further to the centre, they felt around deeper in the abdomen to find the aorta, the large main artery. That, too, had been hit by the bullet. The superior mesenteric artery, the large artery that branches off from the aorta in the upper abdomen to supply the small intestine with blood, had been shot off. Perry closed the hole in the aorta with his finger and clamps were placed around it and on the detached intestinal artery. It was a complete mess, but the loss of blood seemed to have been stemmed for the moment. If you read the operative report, you can feel the relief of the entire surgical team at this point. The patient's blood pressure rose again to an acceptable level.

And yet, they must have known that they stood little chance of saving Oswald's life. The risk of death from acute combined injury to both the inferior vena cava, the body's largest vein, and the aorta, the largest artery, is exceptionally high (more than 60 per cent). That sombre prognosis is of course attributable to the enormous loss of blood from both injuries, from the aorta due to the high pressure and from the hollow vein due to the direct connection to the heart. The difficult access to these hidden structures and the many organs in the immediate vicinity that can also be damaged do not help increase the likelihood of a successful outcome. On the battlefield, where injuries are mainly caused by high-velocity fire, victims with severe damage to the major blood vessels rarely make it to the operating table alive. It is different in the case of civilian bullet wounds, which are mainly caused by handguns, as was the case in Ruby's attack on Oswald.

The anaesthetist during the operation was Dr M. T. Jenkins. The reports state explicitly that the entire procedure was performed without anaesthesia. The patient no longer responded to the pain from the very start, and was therefore only administered pure oxygen. Dr Paul Peters, a surgeon who was present in the operating room, said later in an interview that he recalled three men in green scrubs who clearly did not belong to the operating team. Although Oswald had a breathing tube in his windpipe that would prevent him from speaking, had been unconscious for some time, was on the point of death and had three surgeons poking around in his abdomen, the men still stood at the head end of the table, yelling into his ear, 'Did you do it? Did you do it?' This led Peters to conclude that the authorities had not yet obtained a full confession from the suspect.

The clamps held and the loss of blood seemed under control. A total of nine litres of fluid and sixteen half-litre units of blood were administered. Yet, still the pulse became weaker and slower, and suddenly stopped altogether. This complete absence of a heartbeat is known as asystole or flatline. Was the patient still bleeding somewhere else? In his chest perhaps? Had his heart been hit? The surgeons continued the fight, performing an immediate thoracotomy – making an incision in the left chest cavity between two ribs. They opened the chest, but found no bleeding. Then the pericardium: also no bleeding. Perry, McClelland and Jones took Oswald's heart in their hands in turn to perform open-heart massage, rhythmically squeezing it. As they kept that up for some time, Shires cut out the bullet from just below the skin on the right of the body, as evidence.

Calcium, adrenaline and xylocaine were injected directly into the heart, but to no avail. The heart was by now hardly refilling itself; the circulatory system had practically bled empty. Then the heart started to fibrillate. Instead of contracting rhythmically, the heart muscle made chaotic, uncontrolled movements. The surgeons performed defibrillation, increasing the charge in steps to 750 volts. The heart stopped fibrillating but did not resume beating. Not wanting to give up, they inserted a pacemaker wire, but that too failed to stimulate a strong heartbeat. Jenkins, the anaesthetist, established that the patient no longer responded to stimuli, was no longer breathing independently, and that his pupils no longer contracted when light was shone into them. The surgeons ceased their efforts – Oswald was dead. When they closed up the abdomen and the chest cavity, they were two gauzes short. The operation had lasted eighty-five minutes. The loss of blood was estimated at almost eight and a half litres (a human body contains no more than six litres of blood).

Oswald was not a simple man. He had served in the US Army and had lived in the Soviet Union for several years. Was he a disturbed loner, or did his past suggest secret government activities? Right up to his murder, he himself insisted that he had been framed. He was twenty-four when he died.

But imagine that Perry and his colleagues had been able to save Oswald. They would have kept him in a medically induced coma to improve his chances of survival and, even after that, he would have spent months in intensive care. He might even have needed a number of further operations. He would have been a mental and physical wreck. If he had not succumbed to some complication or other and had eventually left the hospital alive, he would probably have needed a further year's convalescence before he could once again become more or less the same Lee Harvey Oswald as before the shooting. And for what? He would probably have been found guilty anyway and sentenced to death.

Retroperitoneum

Both lungs and the heart are located in a more of less separate cavity, the former in the left and right chest (or thoracic) cavity, and the heart in the pericardium. The largest cavity in our bodies is the abdominal cavity, which contains the stomach, the small intestine, the large intestine (colon) with the appendix and the greater omentum (epiploon), the liver and the gall bladder, the spleen, the womb and the ovaries. The remaining organs in the torso are embedded in fatty or connective tissue, and are therefore not 'loose' in a cavity. They are the oesophagus, the thymus, the major blood vessels, the pancreas, the kidneys, the adrenal glands, the prostate, the bladder and the rectum. The abdomen can be divided into two compartments: the abdominal cavity at the front, and behind it, the retroperitoneum. Located between the abdomen and the back, the retroperitoneum is difficult to get to during surgery. It is deep down in the torso and all the organs in the abdominal cavity are in front of it. And, because the organs in the retroperitoneum are surrounded by fatty and connective tissue, searching for them is like rummaging around in a lucky dip. The retroperitoneum can be accessed through the abdomen of a patient lying on their back, where it then forms the 'floor' of the abdominal cavity. But it can also be accessed from the side, with the patient lying on their side. This is known as a lumbotomy, literally 'an incision in the flank' and is the classic way of accessing the kidneys and the ureters.

24

Prosthesis

Une belle épaule de la belle époque: The Baker Jules Pedoux

SURGERY HAS ALWAYS been about dexterity, but it has also gradually become increasingly dependent on technology. Today, technology is indispensable even for routine operations. The technological revolution in surgery started a century and a half ago and was driven by a small number of hopelessly optimistic surgeons.

Western civilisation had never taken such a great leap forward as at the end of the nineteenth century. The Industrial Revolution was the culmination of the Renaissance, the Enlightenment and many other revolutions that preceded it. It was a period of new ideas, philosophies, discoveries and inventions. There was a widespread sense of optimism. The future belonged to technology. Nowhere was this optimism of the new age as prevalent as in France. There, the new emphasis that emerged in the nineteenth century did not lead to prudishness and grey industrial cities as in England, or to wild lawlessness as in America, but to daring, enjoyment and grandeur. It was the belle époque. And the centre of this 'beautiful era' was of course Paris. Paris had splendid avenues and boulevards, railway stations like palaces, museums, parks and fountains. It was a dazzling city, the city of Maxim's, the Moulin Rouge and the Folies Bergère, of Toulouse-Lautrec, Sarah Bernhardt and the cancan. The most renowned surgeon in this renowned city was Jules-Émile Péan. In 1893, after building his career in the Hôpital Saint Louis, he set up his own hospital on the Rue de la Santé and gave it the less-than-modest name Hôpital International.

The nouveau riche who were having the time of their lives in Paris were, however, in stark contrast to the hard-working labourers in the poor outer districts. Strangely enough, this class distinction was expressed in two chronic infectious diseases that affected all layers of the population: tuberculosis for the poor and syphilis for the decadent 'happy few'. Both diseases were ubiquitous and were partly responsible for the relatively short life expectancy of forty to fifty years of age. For that reason, most people in the nineteenth century did not live long enough to suffer from diseases that typically affect the elderly and which became commonplace in the twentieth century. Osteoarthritis (wear and tear on the joints), for example, was not very common – joints were more commonly affected by tuberculosis or syphilis.

Jules-Émile Péan described a specific case of a shoulder affected by tuberculosis, together with his typical, hopelessly optimistic nineteenth-century solution to the problem. With the assistance of a handy dentist, he replaced the shoulder with a new, mechanical joint. The patient was a poor wretch from the banlieues, a thirty-seven-year-old baker called Jules Pedoux, who had probably contracted tuberculosis as a small boy since there are often decades between the first infection with tuberculosis – which always starts in the lungs – and the development of secondary localisations of the infection elsewhere in the body, such as in the vertebrae or other bones.

Péan's shoulder prosthesis is one of the many wondrous French inventions of the belle époque, on a par with the highest artificial construction in the world (Gustave Eiffel's iron tower), cinematography (the Lumière brothers' film), and the velocipede (Pierre Michaux's bicycle). Amazingly, the artificial shoulder lasted for two years.

Tuberculosis is a disease that, just like syphilis and leprosy, gradually affects the body's tissues and can lead to disfigurement and deformity. They are chronic infections, in other words the symptoms are not usually sudden and severe, but develop slowly, gnawing away at the tissues. That is because they are caused by a specific kind of bacteria – leprosy and tuberculosis by myco-bacteria and syphilis by spirochetes – that invoke a different reaction in the body than most other bacterial infections.

Tuberculosis bacilli attract immune cells that form small clumps of tissue, granulomas, which the bacteria gradually destroy. The bacilli are not very aggressive, but extremely persistent, so that the destructive effect in the long term is much greater than with other infections. They slowly spread through the whole body and remain in hiding for many years. Without tuberculostatics – anti-biotics that specifically combat tuberculosis bacilli – they would never leave the affected tissues. Typical symptoms of tuberculosis are nocturnal sweating and slow emaciation. Tuberculosis does not attack local tissues acutely and severely with pus and a red, painful and warm abscess; the local reaction is much slower, but by no means less severe. It results in the gradual destruction of the affected tissues, which are transformed into a cheese-like substance. A tuberculosis abscess is thus known as a 'cold abscess'.

When Jules Pedoux reported to Péan's hospital, he was very sick and emaciated and had a large cold abscess in his left upper arm. There was probably not much to be seen on the outside, but if you had taken hold of the arm, you would have clearly felt a fluid mass deep below the skin. Every movement of the shoulder must have been painful and his hand was probably congested and swollen, and therefore as difficult to use as the upper arm. Péan initially thought that the only way to save the man's life was by disarticu-lation, amputation of the entire arm by separating it from the shoulder joint. The baker steadfastly refused, preferring to die than live with only one arm. After all, he needed both arms to make his living. Péan took up the challenge, probably against his better judgement. He performed an operation, restricting himself to *nettoyage* ('cleaning up') of the cold abscess. He exposed the bone with a long incision in the upper arm from the top of the shoulder. The upper part of the bone, including the rounded head, was completely affected. Péan cleared away all the Camembert-like bone tissue. The periosteum (the membrane covering the outer surface of the bone), the capsule of the shoulder joint, and the socket all seemed to be intact, leaving a well-defined cavity. After this first operation on 11 March 1893, the patient recovered within a few days and his arm survived.

Péan was familiar with temporary implants of platinum in the faces of patients whose noses and jaws had been deformed by syphilis and tuberculosis. He asked a dentist, a Dr Michaels, to build a mechanical shoulder joint for his patient that would be as inert as possible and guarantee the function of the shoulder joint. Michaels came up with an ingenious contraption that, at least in theory, fulfilled both requirements. He made a rubber ball that he boiled in paraffin for twenty-four hours to harden it. There were two grooves in the surface of the ball, at right angles to each other, in which two platinum rings could move. The horizontal ring was fixed to the shoulder socket of the shoulder blade with two small screws. This enabled the arm to move inwards and outwards (exorotation and endorotation). The movement of the vertical ring enabled the arm to be lifted (abduction). This second ring was fixed to a platinum tube that would replace the top section of the upper arm.

Péan implanted the prosthesis shortly after the first operation, reopening the same incision. It fitted well in the now vacant cavity and he stitched the platinum tube in tightly using catgut thread. Leaving a rubber drain in the arm, he sewed up the skin with horsehair stitches. In his report on the patient's progress, Péan wrote that everything proceeded very well. After twelve days, Pedoux was able to walk around again and was discharged after gaining '35 pounds' in weight. Péan was not more specific about how long Pedoux was in hospital – a few months, half a year perhaps? Although he does describe having to drain an abscess in the wound on four occasions. There is no mention at all of how well the arm functioned, which was after all what the whole operation was for. After Pedoux was discharged, Péan did not see his patient at all for another year. This is in itself remarkable – that a renowned surgeon would allow a simple baker to walk off with an upper arm full of platinum (though this precious metal was not considered very valuable at that time).

Why was he so optimistic about this shoulder prosthesis? Louis Pasteur had already proved thirty years earlier that bacteria were responsible for causing diseases and, ten years earlier, Robert Koch had discovered the bacillus that caused tuberculosis. And yet, Péan could not have known much about the mechanism the human body employs to defend itself against intruding bacteria. We now know that an effective local defence response is only possible in healthy tissues. No matter how well Péan had been able to clean the tissues surrounding the cold abscess, the foreign materials – the rubber ball and the platinum tube – offered bacteria somewhere they could survive out of reach of the body's immune system. The whole undertaking was thus doomed to failure from the start – as would become clear a year later.

In 1897, Péan published a report on the follow-up to the operation. About two years after the surgeon had fitted the pros-thesis, Pedoux came back because he was suffering from a fistula, a hole in the upper arm, which continually leaked pus. Péan had the arm X-rayed – a completely new innovation that had just been invented in Germany. He does not report what he saw on the X-ray, but he decided to remove the prosthesis. He cut the arm open again in the same place and saw that an ossified mantle had formed around the prosthesis. The scar tissue of the original cold abscess had festered and had been transformed into bone

Osteoarthritis

Our bones do not normally come into contact with each other. Their ends, in our joints, are covered with a special kind of tissue, cartilage. Cartilage is the ultimate non-stick material. It is many times smoother than polytetrafluoroethylene (PTFE), better known as Teflon and the smoothest synthetic material ever produced. That makes cartilage an almost irreplaceable tissue in our bodies. Unfortunately, it is also one of the few tissues that cannot heal. Cartilage cells, known as chondrocytes, live without a blood supply. They consequently receive little oxygen and nutrients and have an exceptionally low metabolism. Once cartilage has formed in childhood, the cartilage cells hardly grow or develop any further. Unlike most of the other tissues in our bodies, cartilage is therefore almost unable to regenerate. Dead cartilage cells are not replaced by new ones and, because of the absence of blood vessels, it is almost impossible for scar tissue to form if cartilage is damaged. Wear and tear on cartilage tissue is therefore practically irreversible. It also leads to wear and tear of the joint, which is known as osteoarthritis. It can develop later in life in the weight-bearing joints (knees, hips and ankles) or at a younger age after a fracture or other injury to a joint. Typical symptoms of osteoarthritis are stiffness in the joint, especially in the mornings, and pain at the start of a movement. At a more advanced stage, it can also cause pain at rest and progressive loss of function in the joint. Both problems can only be treated by full or partial replacement of the joint. Metal and Teflon are usually used for artificial joints.

tissue. It was a complete mess, but nevertheless seemed strong enough to ensure that the arm could retain its length, even without the prosthesis. Péan removed the prosthesis, which had probably worked itself loose from all the attachment points anyway. He closed the wound up again and the patient began the recovery process. Again, Péan gave no information about the function of the shoulder or the arm, or whether he had solved the problem of the fistula. Nevertheless, he proudly presented his account of the case to the Académie de Médicine.

Although Péan of course grossly overestimated the success of his treatment, he was certainly ahead of his time. He was, however, not the first surgeon to replace a joint. In 1890 the German Themistocles Glück already had no less than fourteen total joint replacements to his name, including knees, wrists and elbows, all made of ivory. He had even had the various parts of the joints made in different sizes so that he could find the right fit for both sides of the joint during the operation and assemble the two ivory components together on the spot. But Glück, too, had no luck. His patients also suffered from tuberculosis and, like Péan, he did not understand that treating joints affected by bacteria was not the right choice for a pioneer in prosthetics. As we now know, an artificial joint has to be fitted in absolutely sterile conditions. Every bacterium that finds its way onto the prosthesis during the operation will irrevocably lead to the whole thing becoming infected, which can only be treated by removing it again.

When tuberculosis and syphilis were repressed by the discovery of tuberculostatics and antibiotics and people lived longer, a group of patients emerged with a disease that can be treated with artificial joints. Osteoarthritis is wear and tear of a joint, without infection, caused by many years of excess load on the joint. It mostly occurs later in life. Osteoarthritis is ideal for joint replacement. A combination of rubber and ivory proved not to be hard enough. Ivory and wood were tried out, but these natural materials dissolved in the body. Platinum became far too expensive and steel was liable to rust. In 1938, vitallium was introduced in prosthetic surgery. Vitallium is a metallic alloy of cobalt, chromium and molybdenum and is extremely strong and resistant to wear, does not rust, and cannot invoke an allergic reaction. Modern implants are made of titanium or complex alloys combined with Teflon.

Today, following Glück, artificial joints are supplied in various sizes for both sides of the joint and are measured up and assembled during the operation. The individual components are joined to the patient's bone with screws or epoxy cement that is applied as a paste and then hardens. The most common joint replacements are hips, knees and shoulders. The purpose of these operations is firstly to relieve the pain caused by osteoarthritis and secondly to stop the deterioration of the joint function.

With today's knowledge, Péan's prosthesis operation seems to have been completely pointless. The pain was already alleviated by the first operation, which cleaned up the cold abscess. The prosthesis most likely made no difference in that respect. On the contrary, the contraption must have felt uncomfortable, to say the least, among all the muscles of the arm. The third operation showed an advanced degree of ossification in the upper arm. That can only mean that Pedoux must have all but completely lost the use of his shoulder. He could probably hardly move his arm at all and his shoulder may have been frozen. But that would also have happened without Péan's prosthesis. All in all, the contraption did little good, but also little harm.

Péan did leave us with another useful invention. He is responsible for the basic design of nearly all modern surgical clamps and needle holders. It comprises two opposing metal handles for the thumb and index finger, each with a toothed projection. The teeth can be interlocked like a ratchet to hold the clamp shut. Péan was also the first surgeon to remove a spleen, and to make an almost successful attempt to remove part of a stomach. A year after his last report on the baker and his shoulder, Péan contracted pneumonia. He died at the age of sixty-seven. What happened to Jules Pedoux is unknown.

And Michaels's and Péan's surgical masterpiece? Péan initially kept it but, one way or another, Jules Pedoux's artificial shoulder ended up in the hands of an obscure American dentist. He took it with him back to the United States, where it can now be seen in the Smithsonian Institute in Washington DC.

The body can deal remarkably well with foreign materials, as long as no bacteria can get at them. The story of the baker and the history of joint prostheses indeed shows that the acceptance of foreign materials by the body depends on the absence of infection. If bacteria attach to something foreign in our bodies, they are apparently beyond reach of the immune system. Prosthetic material will therefore only be accepted if it is fitted under absolutely sterile conditions. That applies not only to artificial joints, but also to the synthetic textile used to repair hernias, metal clips and staples, pacemakers, synthetic arteries, screws and metal plates for fractured bones, synthetic lenses for the eye, artificial ossicles for the middle ear, drainage systems in the brain, metal stents in blood vessels, mechanical valves in the heart and silicone breast implants.

Sutures are an exception. They cannot always be left behind in the body, which is why absorbable thread is mostly used. If there are bacteria on the sutures, instead of opening up the patient again to retrieve the thread from deep inside the body you can just wait. Once the suture has dissolved, the bacteria will usually give up. Since Roman times, thread made of dried sheep or goat gut was used to stitch up wounds. Péan also mentioned using gut in his report.

25

Stroke

The Neck of Vladimir Ilyich Uljanov: Lenin

'A S FOR YOU, Ilyich,' a simple peasant had once predicted, 'you'll die of a stroke.'

'Why?' Ilyich had asked.

'It's that terribly short neck of yours,' the peasant had explained.

When Vladimir Ilyich Uljanov told this anecdote about himself, he was fifty-two years old and recovering from his second stroke. A few months later, he had another one and, within a year, he was dead. In the many photographs of him, he does have a notably short neck and, in all the thousands of statues of him that used to stand in squares in almost every town and city to the east of the Iron Curtain, his head does seem to be sitting right on top of the collar of his shirt. Nevertheless, a short neck does not heighten the risk of a stroke. So why, after April 1922, did this relatively young man suffer one cerebral infarction after another?

Vladimir Ilyich Uljanov is better known under his revolutionary pseudonym Lenin, leader of the Russian Bolsheviks and of the October Revolution, and father of the Soviet Union. The Soviet media published only praise and positive news on the leaders of the state. When Lenin had his first stroke in May 1922, it reported that he had suffered a stomach infection after eating a rotten fish. The leader had allegedly made a rapid recovery and the months of convalescence that followed were officially referred to as a holiday. However, the stroke could not be kept secret for long

251

and there was much speculation about what had caused it. One suggestion linked the stroke to something that had happened not long previously – Lenin had recently undergone an operation on his neck. That link is indeed striking if you know how a stroke is caused.

The official medical term for a stroke is a cerebrovascular accident (CVA), which means an event affecting the blood vessels in the brain. Worldwide, more than 10 million people a year suffer a stroke. There are two kinds of stroke, a cerebral infarction (ischaemic stroke) and a cerebral haemorrhage (haemorrhagic stroke). A cerebral infarction happens when a blood vessel in the brain becomes blocked. The cause, however, lies outside the brain. If a blood clot forms in the arteries in the neck and then breaks loose, it will flow upwards into the head with the blood and, somewhere deep in the brain, block a small blood vessel. This is known as an embolism and the blood clot as an embolus. In the case of a cerebral haemorrhage, a small blood vessel in the brain bursts of its own accord, flooding the surrounding brain cells with blood. In both cases, the brain tissue is damaged, leading to a sudden loss of brain functions. The lost functions can sometimes recover fully or partially. If the symptoms have completely disappeared within a day, the stroke is referred to as a transient ischaemic attack (TIA), literally a short-lived attack caused by a shortage of oxygen. A TIA can be an indication of a pending real stroke.

The loss of function often takes the form of paralysis of an arm or leg, a drooping mouth, or problems with speaking or comprehending language. Because all connections between the brain and the rest of the body cross sides, a stroke in the left half of the brain will produce symptoms in the right side of the body, and vice versa. Paralysis in an arm and a leg on the same side of the body is known as hemiparesis, literally 'half paralysed'. The parts of the brain that are responsible for speech, comprehending and initiating language are usually in the same half of the brain as that controlling your dominant hand (the one you naturally write with). With people who are naturally right-handed, the area of the brain involved with language is usually in the left half.

A left-sided cerebral infarction can therefore cause a combination of right-sided paralysis and aphasia, the medical term for loss of speech. The embolism originates in the left common carotid artery, the major artery in the neck that feeds the left half of the brain. Lenin was right-handed, and suffered a stroke that caused right-sided paralysis and loss of speech while he was still recovering from an alleged operation on the left side of his neck. That certainly sounded suspicious. Had a surgeon caused his stroke?

What was the reason for the operation? Many of the details of Lenin's health are probably censored, and cult- and myth-forming have added much that is not always true but, between the lines, the Soviet leader did appear to have suffered from a genuine mental disorder. What is clear is that he struggled with headaches, mood changes, a fiery temperament, obsessions, night-mares, and insomnia. Prescriptions have been found in the secret archives in the Kremlin for painkillers and sedatives sent from Germany, including potassium bromide and barbitone, old-fashioned remedies which, if taken excessively or for too long, can cause side effects that are worse than the original complaint.

Lenin was a man who always knew better. Apparently that also applied to the health of his party comrades, as he had made a habit of determining – together with other members of the politburo, the highest party committee – when a comrade was in need of rest. A comrade would then be sent, for his own good and whether he liked it or not, to a health resort or, in the worst case scenario, a psychiatric institution, without a doctor ever being consulted. Now Lenin's own health was on the politburo's agenda. He had changed from an intelligent and impassioned visionary into a cruel and neurotic dictator, and his symptoms were getting worse. In 1921, the other members of the politburo, including Trotsky and Stalin, sent him to his country mansion in Gorki, about an hour's journey to the south of Moscow.

All kinds of doctors visited him and came up with a wide variety of diagnoses. Some of them, including Ivan Pavlov (of Pavlov's dogs fame), claimed that Lenin was suffering from syphilis. Others concluded that it was a purely psychological disorder, such as chronic depression, or 'neurasthenia' – similar to what we would today call 'burnout'. But German medical consultant Professor Georg Klemperer came up with something completely different. He suggested that Lenin's problems were caused by lead poisoning resulting from two bullets that, for many years, had been lodged in his neck.

Some years earlier, several attempts had been made on Lenin's life. In January 1918, his car had been shot at in St Petersburg (which would later be renamed Leningrad), but he was not injured. On 30 August of the same year, a month and a half after the tsar and his entire family had been killed under Lenin's orders, he was severely wounded when a young woman shot at him from close range in Moscow. Fanya Kaplan, twenty-eight, fired three times, hitting Lenin with two bullets, both in the area of his left shoulder.* The third shot hit a bystander, a woman called Popova, in the left elbow. Comrade Lenin lost consciousness and fell to the ground, breaking his left upper arm. He came round quickly, was pulled into his car by his driver, and rushed, bleeding, to his apartment in the Kremlin. There, he

---

* The Soviet reports are not clear. I conclude from them that one bullet was lodged on the left side, deep in the lower part of the neck, where the neck continues into the shoulder region, and that the other got stuck more superficially under the skin above the right joint between the chest-bone and collarbone. There were no exit wounds. It would appear that Lenin was shot from the left side.

walked upstairs to the third floor. Fearing further attacks, he remained within the walls of the Kremlin and doctors did not come to examine him until early on the morning of the following day. Surgeon Vladimir Nikolaevich Rozanov examined him and was seriously alarmed. Lenin was deathly pale, short of breath, had blue lips and his blood pressure was so low that his pulse was no longer detectable. The patient tried to reassure the surgeon and told him in a weak voice not to be concerned, but Rozanov knew better. The situation was serious. He tapped Lenin's chest with his fingers and, instead of hearing a hollow sound, heard a muted sound on the left side. He concluded that the left chest cavity was filled with blood, explaining his patient's pale colour and low blood pressure. That could have compressed the left lung, which would explain the blue lips and the shortage of breath. He could feel a bullet just below the skin, above the joint between the sternum and the right collarbone. The bullet wound was to the left, at the base of the neck. It must somehow have passed through the neck, between the spine, the oesophagus, the windpipe and the blood vessels without having caused much damage. A second bullet had lodged in the area of the left shoulder. Lenin therefore had two bullets in his body, one of which must have caused the bleeding in the upper left of the chest cavity.

The doctors insisted that Lenin should not speak or move and should rest. The immediate danger had passed, otherwise he would not have survived the hours after the attack. He was put to bed, with the broken arm in traction. It was then a matter of waiting. The doctors were concerned that the bullets would cause an infection, but decided to wait and see how that developed. Their weakened patient would probably not survive an operation to remove them, and Lenin himself urged them to leave both bullets where they were. He recovered slowly, there was no infection and, three weeks later, he was able to leave his bed.

Subclavian steal syndrome

A stricture (stenosis) or blockage (occlusion) in an artery as a result of arteriosclerosis can in theory occur anywhere, but usually develops in parts of the body where there is turbulence in the flow of blood. A notable syndrome occurs when a particular large artery becomes blocked in a very specific place. Subclavian steal syndrome is the name given to a blockage of the subclavian artery, the artery below (sub) the collarbone (clavicle), which supplies the arm with blood. The blockage occurs just before the vertebral artery – one of the four arteries to the brain – branches off from the subclavian artery. The two carotid arteries at the front and the two vertebral arteries at the back come together below the brain to form a ring of arteries known as the circle of Willis, named after the doctor and scientist Thomas Willis. With subclavian steal syndrome, the subclavian artery is blocked but the arm still receives blood from the vertebral artery, the blood flowing in the opposite direction. The circle of Willis then supplies blood not only to the brain but also to a whole arm. If the patient exerts a load on the arm, the muscles 'steal' blood from the brain. The reduced supply of blood to the brain causes diminished consciousness. Consequently, someone suffering from subclavian steal syndrome can faint while, for example, using a screwdriver to turn a screw. The occlusion can usually be cleared by percutaneous angioplasty, in other words, pushing open the blood vessel with a small balloon from the inside.

Fanya Kaplan was executed on 4 September after a short interrogation. The incident inspired Lenin and the Bolsheviks to unleash the 'Red Terror', a purging operation during which tens of thousands of 'reactionaries' were tortured and murdered by the Cheka, the secret police.

In the years that followed, Kaplan's two bullets caused no major problems in Lenin's body. But because they were made of lead and had been in there for so long, the German professor had seen them as a possible reason for Lenin's psychological problems, as chronic lead poisoning can affect the nervous system. The idea was presented to Vladimir Rozanov, the same surgeon who had treated Lenin in 1918, but he thought it irresponsible to risk operating purely on the grounds of what he considered a rather far-fetched explanation of the leader's symptoms. Lenin had also had another surgeon called Moritz Borchardt brought in from Berlin, because he clearly did not completely trust his Russian doctors. But Borchardt agreed that operating was a bad idea, calling the very thought *unmöglich* ('impossible'). In Rozanov's memoirs, he describes how he and Borchardt proposed a compromise with their patient. Lenin did not believe that the bullets were the cause of his health problems, but he had had enough of the doctors with their conflicting advice. They agreed that the surgeons would remove the bullet on the right at the bottom of his neck, because it was close to the surface and easy to get at, and leave the one on the left, which was much deeper, where it was. None of this was released to the outside world. Officially, Lenin was to undergo an operation to remove a bullet that had hit him in 1918. That bullet had struck him on the left side of his body. That the bullet was now on the right and that a second bullet would remain in his left side, was not made clear.

First, the surgeons conducted a fluoroscopy, an old-fashioned method that uses X-rays to obtain real-time moving images. They saw that the two bullets had not moved compared with the X-rays made in 1918. Borchardt performed the operation, assisted by Rozanov, at midday on 23 April 1922 in Soldatenkov Hospital in Moscow. It was, according to Rozanov, a simple procedure. The skin was anaesthetised locally with an injection of Novocain and an incision made to expose the bullet, which could then be squeezed out. To prevent infection the operation wound was not stitched up, but filled with a gauze, which was replaced daily until the wound had healed completely, *per secundam*. It was a minor and successful operation and the patient would normally have been able to return home immediately, but Lenin was kept in hospital for one night, much against his will, to be on the safe side. The wound closed up completely after two and a half weeks.

A month after the operation, on 25 May 1922, Lenin suffered his first stroke. He had partial paralysis on his right side and trouble speaking clearly, suggesting that the problem was in his left carotid artery. A few days later, Lenin's blood was tested for syphilis (the Wassermann test) as, in an advanced stage, syphilis can also affect the brain. The test was negative. Lenin himself was convinced that he was incurably sick and in a hopeless situation. He was desperate and, five days after the stroke, asked his comrade Joseph Stalin to bring him poison. The doctors, however, were able to convince him that his prospects were far less bleak than he thought, but in June and July Lenin noticed that the symptoms of paralysis returned briefly while he was walking. He had also become overly sensitive to noise, violin music in particular, and was driving everyone around him to distraction. He spent the summer convalescing in the country in Gorki, picking mushrooms, breeding bees and weaving baskets. He learned to walk again, rested and practised using his right hand. In October, he was back at work in Moscow.

On 16 December, Lenin had his second major stroke, on the same side. He was again partially paralysed, but his speech was much more badly affected. He recovered gradually until, on 9 March 1923, suffered his third stroke in a year. He could no longer speak clearly, had attacks of rage and was confined to a wheelchair. For months, he was under surveillance day and night. He recovered slightly, was able to talk a little and understand what was said to him, but he no longer appeared in public. The following January, he suffered his fourth and final stroke. It proved fatal. He died on 21 January 1924, aged fifty-three.

Is it feasible that Fanya Kaplan's bullet ultimately felled the Soviet leader? According to Rozanov the surgeons had left the bullet near the left carotid artery in place. If his account is correct, the operation to remove a bullet on 23 April 1922 cannot be blamed for the series of strokes that Lenin subsequently suffered. And yet, there has been much criticism of that operation since from commentators and biographers. The theory of the toxic bullets might seem far-fetched, but in the light of the therapeutic options available at the time, Professor Klemperer's decision seems to have been correct. Five possible causes of Lenin's symptoms had been proposed. Of those five, three could still not be treated in the 1920s: syphilis, depression and arteriosclerosis. What his symptoms required in any case was rest, and rest would also be exactly what was required if the workaholic dictator was suffering from neurasthenia or burnout. Lead poisoning was the least likely cause, but was certainly one that could be treated. It was therefore logical both to order the patient to rest and to remove the bullet, but that was all the doctors had to offer at the time.

Normal, healthy arteries are supple and have a smooth inner wall. Arteriosclerosis affects the inner lining of arteries by depositing cholesterol and chalk, causing inflammation. The disease occurs with increasing age, as a consequence of smoking, genetic predisposition, high blood pressure, obesity and high cholesterol levels. The smooth inner wall of the artery becomes irregular and the supple blood vessel becomes inflexible. The resulting progressive narrowing of the artery does not necessarily cause great problems, as the brain receives blood through four arteries in the neck. Therefore narrowing or blockage of one of the major carotid arteries does not always lead to a cerebral infarction, because the other three arteries can take over. An infarction occurs if something breaks free from the inner lining of the artery, an embolus that is carried along in the bloodstream, and becomes stuck further on in a much smaller artery in the brain, blocking the flow of blood. This loosening of a piece of material from the wall of the artery can occur again and again. That is why Lenin had not only one, but a series of strokes, one after the other. If the affected part of the artery could have been removed, his subsequent strokes could have been prevented.

The operation that could have saved Lenin's life, first carried out in 1954, was a great step forward in surgery. Performed in London by surgeons H. H. Eastcott and C. G. Rob, the procedure is called a carotid endarterectomy, which means 'cutting out the inner lining of the large carotid artery'. The procedure entails locating the large carotid artery and placing clamps above and below the affected part. That half of the brain temporarily receives blood from the three other arteries via the circle of Willis. The artery is then cut open lengthways, the affected inner lining is peeled out, and the artery wall is stitched closed again.

The official cause of Lenin's death was arteriosclerosis of the carotid arteries resulting in multiple cerebral infarctions. It was determined at his autopsy, one day after he died on 21 January 1924. That is unusual for a man of only fifty-three, who had never smoked, was not overweight and whose blood pressure was normal. There had been cardiovascular disease in his family, however. Moreover, there are records of an incident in 1921 – before the operation and the strokes – when Lenin had to postpone a speech because he was unable to speak clearly for a short time. That may have been a TIA, a harbinger of his later strokes. What, however, the arteriosclerosis cannot account for are the psychological problems, the headaches, the obsessions and the insomnia that he experienced before the strokes.

If all the official data and reports are correct, neither the bullet nor the operation caused Lenin's death. It is not too late to examine Lenin's left carotid artery and discover whether Lenin underwent an operation deeper in the neck in search of the second bullet. The dictator's embalmed body, ninety years after his death, is on public display in his mausoleum in Red Square and, thanks to a monthly bath in chemicals to combat a persistent fungal infection, is still in reasonable condition. And, all being well, Fanya Kaplan's bullet should still be in there too.

26

Gastrectomy

Cowboys and Surgeons: Frau Thérèse Heller

IN THE EARLY nineteenth century, surgeon Robert Liston was the big hero in London. He was known as 'the fastest knife in the West End'. Speed, an absolute necessity in the time before anaesthesia, was his trademark. Spectators could hardly keep up with his knife and saw. He always had his scalpel in his inside pocket and it is said that he sometimes held it in his mouth when operating so that it was close to hand to make the next incision. As was customary at the time, he had a bundle of thread through the buttonhole of his lapel, ready to tie off spouting blood vessels. And he sometimes also used his teeth to pull his ligatures tight, so as to keep both hands free. Anything not to slow down. Precision was apparently of less importance. He once cut off a patient's testicles while amputating his upper leg. And there was a notorious case when his knife shot out while he was operating and slashed the fingers of his assistant. There was so much blood pouring out of the patient and the assistant's hand that one spectator literally dropped dead from fright. Since both patient and assistant eventually died from gangrene, this must be the only operation on record with a 300 per cent mortality. And yet, Liston was a great surgeon, achieving results that made his contemporaries green with envy. He devised the small 'bulldog' forceps that are still used to clamp small blood vessels temporarily, and large bone cutters, known as Liston shears.

About two hundred years later, surgeons are shocked when

they see the scars of patients operated on in the 1970s and 1980s. A diagonal scar 30, 40 or even 50 centimetres long on the upper-right abdomen is no exception for a regular gall-bladder operation performed before the 1990s. It sometimes seems that the previous generation of surgeons needed an incision big enough to stick their whole head through. For almost every regular abdominal operation, it was the rule rather than the exception to cut the abdomen open with the largest possible incision along the midline – from the point of the sternum all the way down to the pubic bone.

'A big surgeon makes big incisions' was a proud and often-heard statement in those times. With our current knowledge, we can safely say that is complete nonsense. Yet, back then, there would have been plenty of surgeons who thought the opposite: that the younger generation who practised minimally invasive keyhole surgery were cowboys, just as we now consider the big surgeons with their big incisions to be. Every period has its cowboys in the operating room, but in the context of their time, they were heroes.

Frau Thérèse Heller survived an operation to remove a tumour on the outlet of her stomach three months longer than the first man in history to survive the procedure. Today, we would consider both cases a failure. But Theodor Billroth became a hero after treating Heller, while Jules-Émile Péan – who had successfully performed the operation two years earlier – has almost been forgotten. Péan's patient survived less than five days. Both were prominent surgeons at the end of the nineteenth century. Péan, the man who had fitted the baker with a platinum shoulder prosthesis, was a self-confident surgeon in Paris, the cultural capital of the world, while Billroth was the great professor in Vienna, at that time the scientific capital of the world.

A tumour on the stomach outlet was, at that time, one of the most common forms of cancer. Why that is no longer the case is not completely clear, though it may have something to do with the invention of the refrigerator. An important factor in the development of cancer at that precise spot depends on the presence of a specific bacteria. A series of stomach infections caused by eating contaminated food can cause stomach cancer, even at a relatively young age. Improvements in producing and preserving food in the twentieth century probably reduced the incidence of this form of cancer, but in the nineteenth century it was a widespread problem for which surgeons had no solution. Dying from a tumour on the stomach outlet was an inhuman way to meet one's end. With continual pain, vomiting, thirst and starvation, it was a living death, and the surgeon who could operate successfully to relieve such suffering would be an international hero.

In the second half of the nineteenth century the two basic conditions for performing such a dangerous operation were in place: general anaesthesia (first introduced by William Morton in Boston in 1846, see chapter 10) and antisepsis (Joseph Lister, Glasgow,1865, see chapter 11). It must have felt like a race against the clock to the revered professors of the surgical world to be the first to successfully perform this operation, known medically as a distal gastrectomy [removal (-*ectomy*) of the last (*distal*) part of the stomach (*gastr-*)]. Péan's patient survived the operation in April 1879, but not the difficult post-operative phase, despite the surgeon's efforts. This was because Péan was unable to administer the man sufficient fluid, and direct injection of fluid into a vein – what we now call an intravenous drip – was yet to be invented. Péan nevertheless published the results of his 'successful' operation in the *Gazette des hôpitaux* under the title '*De l'ablation des tumeurs de l'estomac par gastrectomy*' (the removal of tumours in the stomach by gastrectomy). Note the plural of tumours, suggesting that Péan was convinced that stomach tumours could now be successfully removed surgically. A year and a half later, Polish surgeon Ludwik Rydigier attempted to perform the operation, but his patient did not even survive the first day.

It was a treacherous operation, seemingly straightforward but in many ways complex. Probably much more complex than surgeons realised at the time. Their publications show that they were mainly concerned with the best method of joining the two loose ends together after removing the tumour, which is not the most difficult part of the procedure – there are three tricky problems lying in wait for the unsuspecting surgeon. Firstly, the outlet of the stomach is located at the intersection of a number of important structures in the abdomen. The vulnerable bile duct, the portal vein, the artery of the duodenum and the pancreas are all very close by. It is difficult enough with a normal, healthy stomach to dissect the stomach free from these surrounding structures without damaging them; a tumour in this already crowded environment makes the job even more complicated. Secondly, the contents of the stomach are as acidic as hydrochloric acid. The tiniest leak in the join between the stomach and the duodenum has a corrosive effect and causes peritonitis. Effective drugs to neutralise gastric acid were not yet available. Thirdly, the duodenum, the next section of the gastrointestinal tract after the stomach, is firmly attached to the back of the abdomen. You then have to be fortunate to bring the ends of the duodenum and the stomach together without too much difficulty.

Billroth's patient was at death's door. Thérèse Heller was forty-three years old. She had been unable to keep any food down for weeks and had been living on sips of soured milk. The tumour could be clearly felt in the emaciated woman's upper abdomen, and was about the size of an apple. Before the operation, Billroth rinsed her stomach with 14(!) litres of lukewarm water and on 29 January 1881 he performed the historic procedure. He became a hero overnight and surgeons still write and speak about him with awe and reverence. His historic distal gastrectomy was a genuine turning point, but not because his patient survived the removal of the tumour. More significant was that she had survived the joining together of the stomach and the intestine for more than ten days, proving that a successful intestinal reconnection was possible. This was an achievement that literally pushed back the frontiers of surgery.

An intestinal join, known medically as an intestinal anastomosis, refers to a connection between intestine and stomach or between two sections of the intestine. As such, it cannot be considered a wound like any other. The unclean contents of the stomach and/ or intestine must be able to continue to pass through the system immediately after the join has been completed, without obstructing the healing of the wound. It was not clear until ten days after the operation whether the body would tolerate this exceptional situation.

Why the ten days? The success of an intestinal anastomosis depends on two phases. Firstly, during the operation, an air- and watertight seal has to be created between the two loose ends. That ensures that the harmful contents of the stomach and intestine remain in the system and cannot enter the abdomen and cause peritonitis. That is purely a matter of surgical technique, choosing the right thread, the right knot, enough stitches (fifty in Billroth's case) and making sure the two ends match. A technically well-executed intestinal join will always stay in place for a few days. But then comes the second phase.

The wound healing process in the patient's tissues must take over from the suture. If the tissues around the stitches die, as can happen with wounds, the suture will tear open, no matter how well the stitches have been placed. But if the tissues remain healthy, the process of wound healing will be activated and seal the connection between the two ends with connective tissue. The sealing of the wound with connective tissue occurs in the first ten days. Once that time has passed, a leak can in theory no longer develop. As with a wound in the skin, where the stitches can be removed after ten days, the stitches in an intestinal join are also superfluous after ten days. But you cannot, of course, open up the abdomen again to take them out. The stitches therefore remain in place for the rest of the patient's life or are made with absorbable thread, which completely disappears within a few months.

After Billroth, all stomach and intestinal operations were suddenly possible: for cancer, infectious diseases, functional disorders and life-threatening obstructions of organs. Gastrointestinal operations soon became the most common procedures performed in general surgery and, in the twentieth century, operations were developed that would have been unthinkable in the hundreds of years before that. The profession of surgeon changed unrecognisably.

With hindsight, however, it must be said that the great Theodor Billroth severely lacked modern surgical insight. The most important criticism would be that he focused on the tumour rather than the patient. The patients of Péan, Rydigier and Billroth were all emaciated and at the end of their tether. That made the operations a lot easier for the surgeons, both technically, as there was almost no fatty tissue in the way, and morally, because doing nothing would condemn their patients to an even more miserable death. We now know, however, that being malnourished is not an advantage at all, but creates an enormous risk of serious complications after an operation. Moreover, it was a complex operation, for which you need to take some basic precautionary measures. For maximum safety, for example, good exposure is required; in other words, not only the tumour, but also the area around it, must be clearly visible. You therefore have to take the time to not only dissect the tumour free, but also the organ on which it is growing and other important nearby structures. Billroth did not do this. On the contrary, he made a horizontal incision in the skin above the tumour, so small that he could not even see that the cancer had spread to the rest of his patient's abdomen. Thérèse died from the metastasis only three months after the operation. Secondly, Billroth had not sufficiently thought out his plan for joining the two loose ends after removing the tumour. He himself said that he had been fortunate in being able to bring the ends of the stomach and the duodenum together without too much tension. But what if that had not been possible? What he *had* taken into account was that the two ends are not the same size. The duodenum is about three centimetres in diameter and the stomach more than six. He eventually needed at least fifty stitches to overcome the discrepancy.

It should therefore be seen as a miracle that Frau Heller survived for another three months. In the years that followed, Billroth performed thirty-four similar operations, with a success rate of less than 50 per cent. And yet, he became world famous. He then abused his position to assert, with no sound arguments to back it up, that surgeons should not attempt operations on the heart or even operate on varicose veins. Billroth's operation, known as Billroth I, was soon replaced by a better method, called Billroth II. The B-II is also a distal gastrectomy but includes a trick that no longer makes it necessary to pull the two ends together. This solution was not devised by Billroth himself, but by his assistant, Viktor von Hacker. A number of disadvantages of the B-II were later solved by a French surgeon called César Roux, who added a second join in the intestine, forming a Y intersection. The distal gastrectomy procedure used today is therefore known in full as the 'Roux-en-Y Billroth II' – a strange name for an operation that is still performed regularly.

Staples

In 1907, Hungarian surgeon Hümér Hültl devised a solution to the problem of intestinal joins (anastomoses). They have to be sewn up stitch for stitch, meaning that the success of the entire join depends on the reliability of each stitch. Hültl believed he could achieve a better seal by completing the anastomosis automatically all in one go. He constructed a heavy stapling machine that could simultaneously insert a whole row of staples in the intestinal tissue. Another Hungarian, Aladár von Petz, refined the concept, producing a less bulky version, which was used in the 1920s, but only in exceptional situations. After the Second World War, surgical staples fell into disuse on this side of the Iron Curtain. However, surgeons in the Eastern bloc continued to use them and the stapling machines were further developed and refined in the Soviet Union. Surgeons in the West did not know that their colleagues in the Eastern bloc were still using them, and those in the East did not know that their Western colleagues did not know. In the 1960s, while visiting Moscow, an American surgeon saw a Soviet stapling machine in a shop window. Unable to believe his eyes, he bought it and took it home. He showed it to an entrepreneur, who adapted it to produce surgical staplers on a large scale under the brand name AutoSuture. They were a worldwide success and, since then, almost no operation on the stomach or intestines is performed without the use of staples.

Although Billroth had done something revolutionary and, in the years that followed, would clearly demonstrate a systematic surgical professionalism, he still practised according to the prevailing tradition of short and sharp operations. All in all, Billroth did not as much herald the start of modern surgery – with which he is so often attributed – as mark the end of 'old' surgery. If great men like Péan and Billroth were the cowboys at the end of the nineteenth century – one with his shoulder prosthesis and the other with his stomach operation – two other men stood for the new order of precision surgery in the early twentieth century: Theodor Kocher in Europe and William Halsted in America.

Theodor Kocher's importance for modern surgery is illustrated by the fact that no other surgeon has given his name to so many surgical terms. There are three Kocher's incisions: the first runs obliquely over the right upper abdomen and is used to access the gall bladder, the second is on the side of the thigh and is used for hip operations, while the third is used for removing a goitre, an enlarged thyroid gland. Also, there are two Kocher manoeuvres, one to replace a dislocated shoulder and the other to free the bend of the duodenum in the abdomen, even a verb to describe the latter procedure: to *kocherise*; a Kocher syndrome, a muscular disorder in children caused by a deficiency of thyroid hormones; a Kocher's point, a location in the skull where a hole has to be drilled to drain cerebrospinal fluid from the brain. Pain shifting from the centre of the abdomen to the right lower abdomen in patients with appendicitis is 'Kocher's sign'. A Kocher table can be wheeled over a patient's legs during an operation, Kocher's forceps are the most well-known clamp in general surgery, and Kocher was the first surgeon to be awarded the Nobel Prize in Physiology or Medicine. In 2009, they even named a crater on the Moon after him.

Kocher's main contribution to surgery was the thyroid operation. Under normal circumstances, the thyroid gland is a small organ in the front of the neck that uses the iodine in our food to produce a hormone that regulates our metabolism. In the case of an iodine deficiency, the thyroid slowly gets bigger in order to keep producing sufficient quantities of the hormone. After a number of years it can take on gigantic proportions. The medical term for this growth is goitre. Fortunately, it does not occur as much today, because bakers add extra iodised salt to their bread, but in the past goitre was particularly common in areas where iodine does not occur very much naturally. Because iodine is mainly present in seawater, iodine deficiency is usually prevalent in countries that are far from the sea and in people living in mountainous areas. It was no coincidence, then, that Kocher was Swiss. Because a badly enlarged thyroid can eventually obstruct the windpipe, a goitre operation was sometimes a matter of life and death. Before Billroth settled in Vienna, he had been a professor in Switzerland. He had tried his hand at resecting goitres, but almost 40 per cent of his patients died, so he stopped performing the operation. Later, Kocher tried it and, by 1895, his precise approach to surgery had reduced the mortality rate to less than 1 per cent.

In the American Wild West, William Halsted was once a cowboy among surgeons. He saved his own sister from bleeding to death while giving birth by administering his own blood to her and, at the age of twenty-nine, when he had only been a surgeon for a year, he performed one of the first gall-bladder operations in America – on his own mother. He was addicted to cocaine, and later to morphine. He sent his shirts to a laundry in Paris, officially because they washed them better but more likely to smuggle narcotics. When he wrote an article on the medical use of cocaine as a local anaesthetic, he was clearly under the influence of the drug at the time, as it started with an unintelligible sentence 118 words long. After meeting Theodor Kocher in Europe, he abandoned his life as a cowboy and became the founder of modern surgical training and surgical scientific research in the United States. He developed various operative methods, including an improved intestinal join, and established the basic principles of cancer surgery. Two operations bear his name, for breast cancer and for inguinal hernia. He devised the mosquito forceps which, like Kocher's forceps, are used by every surgeon on the planet on a daily basis. And it was William Halsted who introduced rubber gloves into surgery. He died in 1922 after an operation on his gall bladder performed by his own students.

Following on from the problem of joining together two pieces of intestine, in the early twentieth century Alexis Carrel showed that blood vessels could be reconnected and the blood continue to flow through them unobstructed. That made operations on blood vessels possible, a precondition for the following revolution, transplantation surgery. In 1954, Joseph Murray performed the first successful kidney transplant, between identical twins, and thirteen years later, Christiaan Barnard completed the first heart transplant at the Groote Schuur Hospital in Cape Town. Lastly, in 1982, Michael Harrison performed an open operation on a foetus in the womb of a pregnant woman, proving that even an unborn child could tolerate an operation and develop further into a full-term foetus. The only structures that cannot (as yet) be repaired surgically are the spinal cord and the optic nerve. All other tissues in our bodies appear to be able to withstand an assault by a surgeon.

27

Anal Fistula

La Grande Opération: King Louis XIV

KING LOUIS XIV of France was intelligent and well spoken, an excellent dancer, sociable, self-confident and gallant, big, strong and athletic, and in the best of health. He loved horse-riding, hunting and waging war and was, in James Brown's words, like a sex machine. The Sun King was married several times, had a series of long-term mistresses and countless brief amorous liaisons. He contracted gonorrhoea at the age of sixteen and one incensed husband whose wife had been sleeping with the king is said to have visited a brothel with the sole intent of giving the monarch syphilis – a goal he did not achieve.

Louis XIV dominated the political arena in Europe in the second half of the seventeenth century. His role reached its high (or low) point in 1713 with the Treaty of Utrecht, when the old power relationships in Europe would disappear for good to make way for new ones. Since then, three language areas (French, German and English) have set the tone. The Netherlands and Spain could only bring up the rearguard. Louis reigned for seventy-two years. His will was law; '*L'état, c'est moi*' he is reputed to have said – 'I am the state'. He was an arch-conservative despot who was responsible for the deaths of hundreds of thousands of soldiers and dissidents. Yet he revolutionised music, architecture, literature and fine art, and surrounded himself with the great creative minds of the Baroque period. His influence apparently extended to a surprising branch of medicine: obstetrics. It is said that through his unpredictable whims Louis XIV literally turned the act of giving birth on its head, although it is doubtful whether that was his intention. At that time, women gave birth as nature intended, squatting on their haunches, so that gravity could give them a helping hand. But Louis could not see the arrival of his bastard child by his mistress Louise de La Vallière clearly enough. So Louise had to lie on her back with her legs open, to give the king a better view – better even than the poor woman herself. Although giving birth lying on your back is difficult and painful, it became fashionable. And women still give birth that way.

He was an exceptional man, if only because he lived to be exceptionally old at a time when few people lived to be old. His son Louis, his grandson Louis and his great-grandson Louis all died before him. Louis XIV died in 1715, four days before his seventy-seventh birthday, of gangrene. His leg was mortified, most likely as a result of hardened arteries, the ageing disease athero-sclerosis. Because his subjects mostly hardly even lived to be forty, the condition was probably unknown. You died before your arteries could go hard. Judging by their treatment the king's physicians had no inkling of what to do about it. They bathed the blackened leg alternately in Burgundy wine and ass's milk. His surgeon Maréchal advised amputation, but the king, tired of life and tired of ruling, refused. He spent his final weeks in terrible pain.

The young Louis XIV had almost died at the age of nine; not so much from the smallpox he contracted, but from the bloodletting administered by his doctors and which had led him to lose consciousness. He did not recover until he recognised his favourite pet, a white pony, which had been dragged up the stairs to his bedside. After that, his health was closely monitored by his personal physicians, who recorded his physical state daily in a *Journal de Santé*. This record was kept faithfully for fifty-nine years, day in, day out, by his doctors Vallot, d'Aquin and Fagon successively. That is how we know that, while on a campaign in 1658, Louis had a fever for so long that it was feared he had malaria, that in all those years he took a bath on at least one occasion, that he was given an enema almost every week for constipation, was short-sighted, was troubled by dizziness and suffered from gout or osteoarthritis. At the age of twenty-five, he had measles and, later in life, was obese, got worms and complained repeatedly of stomach pains. Unfortunately, there is no record of the last four years of his life.

Two other painful episodes for the Sun King are worth mentioning. Louis loved the sweet things in life not only figuratively, but also literally. Sugar was still relatively new in Europe and led to many rotten teeth, particularly among the nobility, who could afford sweet things. Louis had a mouth full of bad teeth and an *arracheur des dents*, a tooth-puller, was regularly summoned to the palace at Versailles to remove yet another royal molar. By the time he was forty, the king had almost no teeth left. This is clear to see in many portraits, on which his cheeks and mouth look like those of an old woman.

On one occasion, things went seriously wrong. The tooth-puller not only had a rotten tooth in his pliers, but a piece of the king's upper jaw, with part of his palate attached to it. What happened to the unfortunate dentist is unknown, but the king developed a severe infection and an abscess in the bone of his upper jaw. The rotten tooth itself could, of course, have caused the abscess. Then it is possible that a piece of infected bone could break loose along with the tooth. In that case, the dentist could do nothing about it. In any case, Louis was in a bad way and there were fears for his life. Several surgeons were summoned. They eventually broke the jaw open further to release the pus and seared the remainder of the cavity caused by the abscess with a branding iron – with the king sitting upright in a chair and without anaesthesia.

One of them would have stood behind the king to hold his head firmly with both hands, perhaps by pressing it against the back of the chair, with the right hand on the forehead and the left on the lower jaw. In that way, he could also force the mouth open. A second surgeon would have stood to one side and pulled the top lip out of the way with both hands to ensure a good view of the upper jaw. A third would be at the fireplace, warming up the branding iron. From his perilous and constrained position, the king must have been frightened to death when he saw the red-hot iron approaching him. The heat in his mouth, the stinking smoke and the excruciating pain must have taken his breath away, but Louis bravely endured the ordeal and soon recovered. He was left, however, with a hole in his palate between his oral and nasal cavities. That caused soup and wine to pour out of his nose when he drank. When he was eating, he could be heard from out in the corridor.

The king was in the habit of receiving his guests while sitting on his *chaise percée*, his commode. Consequently, during an audience or while consulting his advisers, Louis could be defecating in public. There was a junior noble at the court whose only task was to wipe the royal *derrière*. The king never did that himself. Whether it was because of these extraordinary toilet rituals, too much horse-riding, certain sexual preferences, the more than 2,000 documented colonic rinses and enemas his rectum had endured, or perhaps worms in his bowels is not clear but, on 15 January 1686, Louis developed a swelling near his anus. On 18 February, it proved to be an abscess, which burst on 2 May forming a fistula that, despite warm compresses and more enemas, refused to close up.

The word fistula is Latin for tube, pipe or flute. An anal fistula is known as a perianal fistula, meaning a 'fistula in the area of the anus'. It is essentially a small passage, a hollow tunnel, between the intestines and the skin, as though a small creature has gnawed its way out of the rectum to the outside. However it is not caused by small creatures but by bacteria.

A perianal fistula always starts with a small wound in the mucus membrane of the rectum, on the inside of the anus. The countless bacteria in the faeces can cause the wound to become infected. The infection can then become an abscess and, as is the case with abscesses, pus will form and exert pressure on the surrounding area. Around the rectum, the tissues close to the bowel are much tougher than those further away. An abscess adjacent to the rectum therefore tends to move away from the bowel; it burrows through the softer tissues and eventually becomes an abscess below the skin.

The more pus develops in the perianal abscess, the greater the pressure. The patient suffers severe pain and fever. That is what Louis must have experienced in March or April of that year. Eventually, the skin will come under such pressure that it bursts, releasing all its stinking pus. That happened to the king early in May. The pressure then recedes, the fever retreats and the pain stops, but the passage from the small wound in the rectal mucus membrane to the skin almost never heals up on its own, but leaves a persistent fistula.

Why a perianal abscess leaves a tunnel that refuses to heal by itself is not entirely clear. Perhaps the large quantities of bacteria continually present in the rectum or the mucus permanently produced in the mucus membrane have something to do with it. A fistula can stay dormant for a long time, without causing any symptoms or discomfort, but the passage can fill with pus and form a new abscess at any time. That means that once you have suffered from a perianal abscess, there is a great chance of it recurring. In some cases, the tunnel in the fistula can become so wide that bowel gases and even faeces can be released through it, which can of course be troublesome because you have no control over it. That was probably what was causing the king so much discomfort, since a fistula does not necessarily generate many symptoms.

It is important when treating a perianal fistula to distinguish between two types. If the internal wound is very low in the rectum, close to the anus, the fistula tunnel comes out below the anal sphincter. Imagine that you insert a thin rod through the tunnel, from the hole in the skin on the outside to the hole in the mucus membrane on the inside and then cut the tunnel open down to the rod, from one hole to the other. In that way, you open the tunnel up along its whole length, so that the two small wounds at each end of the fistula become one large 'regular' wound. That one open wound can then heal, because the fistula is no longer there. You leave the wound open rather than stitching it up, rinse it six times a day with plenty of water, and wait. After six weeks everything has healed up *per secundam*. This procedure is known as a fistulotomy (a cut of the fistula) or, more graphically, as the 'lay-open' technique. The rod used to find the fistula tunnel is called a probe, as it 'probes' its way through the fistula.

If, however, the internal wound is higher up in the rectum, further inside when seen from the anus, the fistula tunnel can pass above the anal sphincter, or even through it. If you then perform a fistulotomy, you not only cut open the fistula, but also the anal sphincter. That of course has to be avoided as, if your anal sphincter is damaged, you cannot control your bowel movements.

Louis XIV clearly had so much discomfort from his fistula a surgeon was eventually summoned to perform a fistulotomy. However, the surgeon, Charles-François Félix de Tassy, had never performed the operation before. He asked the king for six months to prepare and practised on seventy-five 'regular' patients before cutting open Louis's fistula at seven o'clock in the morning of 18 November 1686. The monarch lay on his stomach in bed, with his legs spread wide and a cushion under his belly. Also present were his wife Madame de Maintenon, his son the Dauphin, his confessor Père François de la Chaise, his physician Antoine d'Aquin and his prime minister, the Marquis de Louvois, who held his hand.

The surgeon had made two instruments for the operation, an enormous anal retractor and an ingenious, sickle-shaped knife – a scalpel with a semicircular probe on its end. That enabled him to probe and cut open the fistula tunnel with the same circular movement. He therefore combined the two tools required for a fistulotomy, the probe and the knife, in a single instrument. De Tassy first spread the king's buttocks, which were substantial, as Louis was by no means thin. That enabled him to examine exactly where the external wound was located – how far from the anus, in front of or behind it, and to the left or right. He then inserted his finger into the royal aperture to feel the internal opening, if there was one to feel. So far, the king would have felt no pain, only discomfort and embarrassment. The surgeon would then have asked the patient to lie still while he inserted the retractor and slowly screwed it open. With a little luck and enough light, the internal opening in the rectum should now have been visible. The spectators may quite possibly have taken a look over the surgeon's shoulders at this point.

Now the surgeon had to warn the king that it was going to hurt, but that he had to lie still for a short while longer. De Tassy inserted his 'fistula probe-cum-knife' into the external opening and pushed it inwards, gently but firmly, until he came to the internal opening. That was painful. Everyone had drops of sweat on their foreheads, and hoped that it would not last too long. When de Tassy saw the probe come out of the internal opening, he knew that, as far as he was concerned at least, the hard part was over. But, for the unfortunate patient, the worst was yet to come. With a short, sharp yank, the surgeon pulled the knife through the fistula. The king figuratively clenched his

Haemorrhoids

A lot can go wrong in and around the anus. The branch of medicine that deals with such problems is known as proctology. Proctological surgery includes the treatment of perianal fistulas and abscesses, anal warts and tumours, anal fissures, prolapses, anal incontinence and haemorrhoids (piles). Haemorrhoids are varicose veins in the three veins of the anus. From the perspective of someone lying on their back with their legs pulled up, these three veins are located at five o'clock, seven o'clock and eleven o'clock, i.e. rear left, rear right and front right. Haemorrhoids mostly cause no problems at all, except for itching and a little loss of blood. But if the flow of blood through the varicose vein is obstructed, it can generate quite sudden and severe pain. This can occur, for example, after sitting on a plane for too long. Napoleon Bonaparte allegedly lost the Battle of Waterloo because of this problem. If the symptoms become chronic, a haemorrhoidectomy – surgical removal – may be necessary. They can also be tied with elastic bands (Barron ligation), shrunk by means of an injection (sclerotherapy), or seared using electrocoagulation. In the Middle Ages, this was done using a glowing copper staff stuck through a cold lead pipe placed on the pile. Newspapers play an important role in the development of haemorrhoids: if you take a newspaper, comic, smartphone or laptop with you to the toilet, the pressure in the veins of the anus will be too high for too long. So don't sit there any longer than you need to!

teeth, but did not cry out. The fistula was cut open. De Tassy quickly removed the large retractor from the anus and stemmed the bleeding with a wad of bandages. The patient would have felt a small stream of blood flow down his legs, but that soon stopped, too.

Louis left his bed after a month and was back on his horse

three months later. He was not ashamed of his anal problem. The whole of France knew about it and had shared their monarch's anxiety in the weeks of waiting. Fortunately, the king survived, proving that the operation had been a success. Wearing bandages in one's trousers even became the fashion for a short time at the court in Versailles, in imitation of the brave king. The fistulotomy became known as *La Grande Opération* or *La Royale*. The story goes that Félix de Tassy was asked by at least thirty courtiers to perform the same operation, but had to disappoint them, as none of them were actually suffering from a fistula. In January 1687, court composer Jean-Baptiste Lully performed the magnificent *Te Deum* in honour of the king's recovery (that was when he hit his big toe with the conductor's staff).

Given the favourable outcome of the operation and that there was no mention later of the king suffering from incontinence, he must have been suffering from a 'low' fistula, meaning that his anal sphincter was probably spared. Félix de Tassy was fortunate in only having to perform a simple fistulotomy. But how are higher fistulas treated?

Hippocrates already had a solution to that problem more than 2,000 years ago. He was the first to mention the seton method, using a simple thread, in the fifth century BC. The Greek physician described a probe of pliable tin with an eye, like that in a needle, at the trailing end. He passed a thread made of a few strands of flax with a horsehair wound around them through the eye. He first inserted his index finger into the patient's anus and then the probe into the external opening of the fistula. He pushed the probe through the fistula tunnel until he felt it emerge into the rectum with his index finger. He then bent the probe, pulling it out through the anus. With the thread now passing through the fistula to the rectum and out again through the anus, the two ends were tied together.

The thread through the fistula served first to keep the tunnel open, so that any pus that formed in it could drain out by running down the thread. That stopped an abscess developing or recurring. The thread was then tied more tightly so that, in the days and weeks that followed, it would gradually dig its way through the tissues of the anal sphincter. So slowly, that the damaged muscle fibres behind the thread would have time to heal again. It was a fistulotomy in slow motion, which spared the anal sphincter. The cutting effect of Hippocrates's thread was mainly due to the coarse flax, but that could break prematurely. That was the reason for the horsehair: you could use it to pull a new flax thread through the fistula without having to use the tin probe again.

Today, a wide range of methods are tried out to treat high anal fistulas; for example, by filling them up with various substances or sealing them off with mucus membrane. But the most commonly used method remains Hippocrates's classical seton stitch, a simple thread that slowly cuts through tissues. Synthetic materials and elastic are used rather than flax and horsehair, but the effect is the same and, in many cases, the results are satisfactory.

Félix de Tassy had thus obviously not learned his procedure from the books of Hippocrates, as he used a knife rather than a thread on the king's fistula. He may have read about this method in the work of successful English fistula surgeon John Arderne of Newark-on-Trent. Arderne wrote a handbook on fistulas in 1376, with illustrations of his operational methods and the instruments he had made himself. Arderne treated all fistulas with a straightforward fistulotomy, nothing fancy. And yet he achieved much better results than his colleagues. His fame was probably due to the mildness of his post-operative care, which enabled the cut-open fistulas to heal much better than those operated on by his fellow surgeons. He stemmed the flow of blood from the wound with a piece of cloth rather than with a branding iron and had the wound cleaned with water rather than with corrosive salves and administering enemas. Louis XIV, too, benefited from this milder approach.

Arderne had been a military surgeon in the Hundred Years' War, where he had seen a large number of knights suffering from fistulas. In their heavy armour, they bumped up and down in the saddles of their horses, while the sweat from their exertions, fear and heat ran down their backs and into the crack between their buttocks. The continual irritation led to an abscess near the coccyx, which burst open, leaving a hole that looked like a perianal fistula.

It proved, however, to have been something different. Exactly the same problem that John Arderne had encountered among knights bumping up and down in their saddles in the fourteenth century recurred some six hundred years later in a different war, again among soldiers bumping up and down on their coccyxes. This time they were not knights on horseback, but soldiers in jeeps in the Second World War. The jeep was designed for rough terrain, but had hard seats and no suspension. Tens of thousands of American soldiers spent weeks on end in hospital being treated for abscesses between their buttocks.

In such cases the infection, known as a pilonidal cyst, originates a little higher than with a perianal abscess and does not start in the rectum. The cause is not completely clear, but it always occurs in the same place, the spot where we no longer have a tail. Where our tails would have been, a small area remains after birth where the supply of blood to the subcutaneous tissue is less than ideal and there is more chance of hair growth under the skin. Some people have a small dimple in the skin at this spot. The subcutaneous hair can cause a pus-filled infection, especially if the area is continually irritated, as with the soldiers in their jeeps. For that reason, an infected pilonidal cyst is also known as 'jeep seat' or 'jeep riders' disease'.

John Arderne had not noticed that the knights' abscesses were different from real perianal fistulas, and the distinction was not made in the seventeenth century either. King Louis, however, was certainly not suffering from a pilonidal cyst. A pilonidal cyst is not an open-ended tunnel (a fistula) but a dead end (sinus) through which Félix de Tassy would never have been able to pull his specially designed 'fistula probe-cum-knife'. Both complaints are more common in men than women, and perianal fistulas mostly develop at a slightly later age – between thirty and fifty – than pilonidal cysts. Louis was forty-eight. Perianal fistulas can sometimes be caused by Crohn's disease, inflammation of the bowel, but the cause is mostly unclear. In Louis's case, the unhygienic conditions at Versailles may have played a part. Due to a lack of clean water and refrigerators, people living at the court had just as much chance as everybody else of suffering regularly from diarrhoea, caused by food poisoning. Moreover, the Sun King did not wash. He smelled so badly that once, when being visited by an ambassador, he was friendly enough to open a window himself so that his guest was not offended by his bodily odour.

Surgeon Félix de Tassy never took up the knife again after operating on the king, a fact blamed on the stress, which had allegedly become too much for him, though the generous pension, the country estate and the title he received for the operation probably had more to do with it. His 'fistula probe-cum-knife' can currently be seen in the Musée d'Histoire de la Médecine in Paris.

At that time surgery was not considered an honourable profession. But that was going to change. The whole of Europe heard about the royal fistulotomy. Songs and jokes appeared making fun of Louis's fistula. Everyone was talking about it. The success of the fistulotomy exposed the lack of proficiency of doctors with their purgatives, rinses, potions and bloodletting. In the century after the royal operation, the popularity of surgeons reached unprecedented heights.

28

Electricity

600 Volts: The Electric Eel at Artis Zoo

SURGEONS WORK WITH electricity on a daily basis. Depending on the voltage, conductivity and frequency, electricity can be harmless, useful, obstructive, dangerous or lethal. On 1 March 2013, an extraordinary operation was performed in Amsterdam that clearly showed the dangers of electricity. But, the operation was not performed by a surgeon and the operating room was not in a hospital. The location was Artis Zoo and the procedure was performed by Marno Wolters, a vet who operates on a wide variety of animals.

Surgeons, of course, restrict themselves to mammals, more specifically to one species of primate, but most operations performed on Homo sapiens can also be carried out on other animals and developments in surgery help advance veterinary medicine. Neutering and spaying operations are part of a vet's daily work, but they also perform caesarean sections on dogs, stomach operations on cows and tummy tucks on pot-bellied pigs. They repair abdominal hernias on horses, fix fractured bones on cheetahs and perform dental corrections on hippopotami.

There are surgeons who operate on the tiny stomachs and bowels in mice in the context of their scientific research, but it would be especially interesting to perform, say, an oesophageal operation on a flamingo, angioplasty on the carotid arteries in a giraffe's neck, a pulmonary operation on a turtle, an appendectomy on a koala bear (whose appendix is two metres long), or operate on a tiger's thyroid gland, if that were possible. How about open-heart surgery on a whale (whose heart is big enough to stand in) or a nose correction on an elephant?

The operation at Artis Zoo was no less remarkable and, with this animal, it was dangerous too. Wolters performed his operation on an *Electrophorus electricus*, an electric eel. The animal, which had been swimming in the aquarium at the zoo for many years, had developed a swelling in its abdomen. Electric eels are fish around one and a half metres long that have the ability to generate electric shocks, making them more dangerous than a live electric socket under water.

There is nothing extraordinary about an animal that can generate electricity. Every cell in the body continually creates an electrical field between its interior and the outside world. The voltages generated in our own bodies are very weak, but are strong enough to be easily measured. We can measure the electrical impulse of the brain, for example, with electroencephalography (EEG) or of the heart with electrocardiography (ECG). Nerve cells use their electrical charge to transfer signals. Our brains are an enormous regulatory centre that runs on electricity. A lot of energy is required to generate and maintain all that electricity. About a fifth of all the oxygen we need goes to our brains to supply the necessary electrical power.

The organs that an electric eel uses to generate electricity are unique. Rather than producing their electrical charges individually, they generate it in series, so that the power of the charge is cumulative. This enables the eels to produce very high voltages. As they need large quantities of oxygen to generate all this electricity, much more than a fish can extract from the water through its gills, electric eels have to come to the surface regularly to inhale extra oxygen from the air.

An electric eel has three organs that generate electricity. All three are in its tail, which accounts for almost the whole length of the fish. The Sachs' organ emits weak electrical impulses that the fish uses as a sort of radar to feel its way through its surroundings (its eyes are very small). It is used to locate prey, which can then be paralysed by an electrical charge from the Hunter's organ. The third, 'main' organ is used when the fish is in danger. It can generate a charge of 600 volts, which can immobilise any animal in the vicinity, including humans.

The abdomen of the electric eel at Artis had been swollen for several weeks and was pushing its head upwards. An electric eel's abdomen is normally small and hardly noticeable between the head and the enormous electrical tail. Initially, the vets at the zoo thought the fish was overeating or was constipated, but reducing its food intake and administering laxatives did not help. Antibiotics also had no effect, so it was probably not an infection. It looked as though the fish had cancer. Its suffering was clearly increasing rapidly and the vets decided to examine it and see if anything could be done. That meant removing the fish from its tank, taking an X-ray and conducting a biopsy – surgically removing a small piece of the swelling and examining it under a microscope. The electric eel would obviously see all this as a threat and would use its 600-volt charges against the keepers. That would exhaust it and it would need extra oxygen. All in all, it was a risky undertaking not only for the humans, but also for the fish itself. The operation therefore had to be carefully prepared.

It was not the first operation on an electric eel. Artis contacted vets in Chicago who had performed the same procedure in 2010. Preparations were made and summarised in a log. It was important to know that an electric eel only emits an electrical charge when it wants to, so never unconsciously. That meant that it would not emit charges if it was asleep – and that had two advantages. Once the fish was under anaesthesia, the operation could be performed without fear of electric shocks. Secondly, the depth of the sleep could be measured simply with a voltmeter in the water. The weaker the charge, the better the anaesthetic was working.

The operation was performed in the gallery behind the large hall of the zoo's historical aquarium. Everyone wore special electrician's gloves, the two keepers responsible for catching and moving the fish even wore rubber diving suits, and the operating table was made from a piece of PVC guttering, in which the fish could be laid for the X-ray and the biopsy. Using a net, the fish was transferred to a plastic tank full of water, through which extra air was pumped. The electric shocks were measured with a simple voltmeter, while the anaesthetic (Tricaine) was added to the water. Over the course of an hour, the intensity of the shocks diminished and the fish's movements decreased.

Once it was fully asleep, it was lifted out of the water and placed in the gully-shaped operating table. The voltmeter showed no more electric charges. The fish's mouth was continually rinsed with the Tricaine solution. The size of the swelling was now clearly visible and hard lumps could be felt in the swollen belly. An X-ray was taken and, wearing his rubber gloves, Wolters made a small incision in the skin above the tumour. An electric eel does not have scales, but skin similar to that of a real eel, which made Wolters's job easier. He removed a small piece of tissue from the abdomen and stitched the wound up with absorbable thread. With fish, it is important to use a suture that does not dissolve too quickly. A wound will heal within two weeks in a warm-blooded animal but fish, which are cold-blooded, have a much slower metabolism. So a suture has to remain in place for six to eight weeks to ensure that the wound heals properly. After the small operation, the fish was placed in a tank of fresh water to come around. It soon started to move again and the first shocks immediately registered high voltages.

Around an hour later, however, there was clearly something wrong with the electric eel. The shocks were no longer regular and it became less active. Then, suddenly, it emitted a single high-voltage electrical discharge and stopped moving completely. The fish was dead. It was as though it had exhaled its final breath in the form of electricity. Had the anaesthesia and the operation been too stressful, or had the cancerous tumour proved too great a burden for it to endure?

Sutures

Sutures are performed using a special tool called a needle holder, in which the needle is tightly clamped. A right-handed surgeon holds the needle holder with the thumb and ring finger of his right hand. In his left hand, he holds tweezer-like forceps to lift the tissue and take the needle over from the needle holder. Suture needles are curved, so that the tissue is manipulated as little as possible during stitching. They are disposable needles to which the suture thread is already attached. The needle and thread come in double-layered sterilised packaging. The outer layer can be opened without touching the inner layer. The operating surgeon or his assistant can then take hold of the inner packaging without touching the outer layer. This ensures that no bacteria are passed on when the surgeon is handed the needle. There are sharp needles, blunt needles, cutting needles, and large and small needles. There are absorbable and non-absorbable suture threads, threads made of one piece and others that consist of several threads woven together. All of these combinations of different threads and needles are packaged separately and with threads of different thickness and strength. The strength of the thread is expressed with a number. Number 1 is quite thick, 2 is very thick, and so on up to 5. A 0 thread is finer, but most threads are even thinner. They are indicated by a series of zeros. Two-zero thread (00) is thinner than 0. Three zeros (000) is a normal thickness for a skin suture. Blood vessels are stitched using very thin six-zero thread while threads with 12 zeros – thinner than a human hair – are used in microsurgery.

Wolters conducted an autopsy on the cadaver. The tumour was gigantic and had spread to the liver and the spleen. Microscopic tests later showed that it was metastatic pancreatic cancer. That explained the rapid growth of the tumour. The fish's prospects would have been very bleak, in any case. Perhaps, by dying after the anaesthesia, it had been spared a lot of suffering.

The electricity that Wolters and his team had to take into account was unpredictable. Surgeons (who operate on people) also have to be aware of the dangers of electricity in their daily work, but fortunately the amount of electricity in an operating room can be regulated and controlled. Electricity is present everywhere during an operation. The anaesthetist's respiratory machine and the instruments that monitor the heartbeat, oxygen level and blood pressure run on electricity. The operating table needs electricity to move, the lights are of course electric, the equipment used for keyhole surgery depends on electricity, the mobile X-ray machines produce kilovolts of electrical charge, and there are computers in the operating room to record and retrieve medical data and video monitors to watch procedures and look at X-ray photographs – all of which are electrically driven. And there are also some operative methods that require electricity, much closer to the patient and the operating staff than you might expect in such a safe situation. For example, almost no operation can be performed in modern surgery without electrocoagulation. This is applied using a kind of electrical knife evolved from a combination of a scalpel and a branding iron. During electrocoagulation, the patient is literally 'live'. And yet it is safe.

In the Stone Age, surgeons used stones. Abraham of Ur used a stone knife to perform circumcisions. The Greeks used scalpels of bronze, the Romans used iron and we use steel. In the past hundred years, thanks to technological developments, new types of knife have been devised. Piezoelectricity (well known from the sonar systems in submarines) is applied during operations in a special instrument that uses vibration to dissect and to stem bleeding. Not long after the power of radiation (nuclear power) had been harnessed, gamma rays were used in surgery with a tool known as a gamma knife. Shortly after the development of usable microwaves (e.g. for cooking), the technique was also introduced in surgery, and the same applies to lasers. But the most successful instrument of all remains the simple electric scalpel, which was introduced into surgery shortly after the widespread introduction of electricity into daily life (the electric light bulb).

Experiments with using electric filaments to stem surgical bleeding by cauterisation (known as electrocauterisation, from the Latin word *cauterium*, branding iron) were conducted as early as 1875. The filament was, however, much too hot and cauterised the surrounding tissues in a much wider area than was intended. It was slow and imprecise, not to mention dangerous.

French physicist Jacques-Arsène d'Arsonval went a step further. He knew that electricity mainly generated heat at the point of greatest resistance. The human body is large enough to conduct electricity without much resistance and it could also flow freely through the metal of the scalpel. The point of greatest resistance was therefore where the scalpel and the body came into contact, more specifically in the small zone of tissues around the tip of the electric knife, exactly where the heat was required for the surgical effect. Moreover, the heat was only generated when there was contact between the scalpel and the tissues.

D'Arsonval came up with the idea that the power of the electric current, which is harmful to the body, could be kept at a low level if the energy were transferred in the form of alternating rather than direct current. Alternating current (AC) is the kind of electricity that comes out of our wall sockets. It is in principle lethal, having a paralysing effect on the nerves, the heart and the muscles. But the French physicist discovered that the undesirable effects of the alternating current disappears if the frequency is sufficiently increased, to above 10,000 hertz.

An electric knife is connected to a generator with a wire. The generator then has to be connected to the patient with a second wire, to complete the electric circuit. The patient thus becomes part of the circuit. Today, that second wire is connected to the patient by means of a conductive disposable adhesive pad attached to the thigh, generally called the 'patient plate'. A surgeon will therefore never start an operation until he has asked the operation team if 'the plate has been attached'.

Heat stems the flow of blood by converting the proteins in the blood and in the surrounding tissues from liquid to solid, just as the white of an egg solidifies when it is boiled. This specific property of protein is known as coagulation. When you do this with electricity, it is called electrocoagulation. If the temperature is increased by applying even more heat to a small area of tissues, all the water in the cells will evaporate suddenly, causing them to explode before the proteins have had the chance to coagulate. The effect is not to stem the bleeding but to cut the tissues.

In the 1920s, American engineer William Bovie further elaborated on the principle of electrocoagulation. He developed a generator in which the level of energy in the tissues could be much better regulated. He achieved that by increasing the frequency of the alternating current to as high as 300,000 hertz. His generator supplied this current in pulses, in what is known as modulated alternating current. Moreover, he could regulate the voltage. A higher voltage was compensated for by reducing the number of pulses per minute, so that the total energy level did not rise too high. This enabled the effect of the heat applied to vary from coagulation to cutting, while the current remained within safe limits. This principle continues to be applied unchanged in surgery today and, in many countries, the electrosurgical device is still called 'the Bovie' after its inventor.

Bovie's instrument was introduced into surgery by Harvey Cushing – the pioneer of neurosurgery – in Boston on 1 October 1926. Cushing focused on the one organ in the human body in which bleeding cannot be stemmed simply by applying pressure, stitching or tying off: the brain.

The brain and most tumours in the head are amply supplied with blood by small blood vessels. Consequently, removing brain tumours proved to be an extremely bloody operation. Cushing developed a number of precautionary measures to deal with that. He used small silver clips that he could attach to small blood vessels to stop them bleeding and which could be left behind in the tissues. Cushing also made a habit of removing brain tumours in sections. If he was forced to stop operating because of excessive loss of blood, he would continue the procedure some days or weeks later when the patient's blood levels had recovered. This was known as the piecemeal method. With major operations, he would ask a volunteer to be present in the operating theatre to donate blood for the patient on the spot if necessary. Mostly, they would be medical students who would take the opportunity to observe the pioneering brain operations close up.

Cushing described the operation in which he used electro-coagulation for the first time in a medical journal, to publicise the importance of this new method of stemming bleeding. He was, however, by no means the first to apply the new technique. Several surgeons had preceded him, but Cushing's application of electrocoagulation in neurosurgery was so successful and Cushing himself was so famous that the publication of the astounding results of that one operation in 1926 proved decisive in advancing the use of the method.

But first a serious problem had to be solved before electro-coagulation could be used more widely. Although the city of Boston was already using alternating current to light streets and houses, the Brigham Hospital, where Cushing worked, still ran on direct current. The operating room therefore had to be connected to alternating current especially for Cushing's groundbreaking operation by running a wire up from the street.

On that day, Cushing used William Bovie's generator to operate on a man with a malignant tumour of the skull, an extracranial sarcoma. He had been forced to suspend his operation on the man three days earlier because of excessive loss of blood. Cushing had not made any great effort to understand the physics behind the coagulation device, saying, 'One may learn to pilot a motor driven vehicle without necessarily knowing the principles of the internal combustion engine.' He had therefore asked Bovie to be present in the operating room in person. If Cushing needed to regulate the amount of current applied to stem the bleeding, Bovie could fiddle with the knobs to give him more or less voltage and more or fewer pulses. Cushing reopened the wound from the first operation and continued removing the tumour piece by piece. This time, rather than using scalpel and scissors, he used electrocoagulation. The smell of the smoke as he cauter-ised the tumour was so bad that spectators in the gallery became nauseous. The medical student waiting to give blood fainted and fell off his chair, but Cushing was immediately convinced: the method was astounding.

During the next operation, to remove a similar tumour from the skull of a twelve-year-old girl, Cushing was able, with Bovie's assis-tance, to remove the tumour completely in one session. Both patients recovered well without complications and Cushing continued to use the Bovie device in all of his subsequent operations. It even enabled him to perform operations that he had previously never dared to undertake. 'I am succeeding in doing things inside the head that I never thought it would be possible to do,' he wrote to a colleague. Surgeons from a wide variety of disciplines all over the world started to follow his example.

At first, things would still sometimes go wrong. During one operation on the skull, a blue flame shot out of the patient's opened frontal sinus. A spark from the electrocoagulation had ignited the flammable ether that the patient was inhaling as an anaesthetic and that had escaped through the surgical opening. After that, Cushing ensured that the anaesthetic was administered rectally rather than through inhalation. On another occasion, Cushing received a shock from a metal wound retractor that he inadvertently leaned on with his arm. That inspired him to use wooden instruments and a wooden operating table for a while, until Bovie found a better solution by adjusting the settings on his generator.

Today, a wide variety of measures are taken to protect patient and operating team from electric shocks. The team wear surgical rubber gloves and the patient, operating table and all electrical equipment are earthed. The whole operating room is a Faraday cage: there is a network of copper wires in the walls and doors to ensure that electrical charges from outside, such as a lightning strike or an overload on the power grid, cannot enter the room and disrupt the operation. Moreover, modern operation complexes are isolated from the outside world. In other words, not a single electrically conductive wire may lead to them directly: the electrical circuits used in the operating room are all supplied through transformers and the data in the computer network is transmitted through fibre-optic cables.

Bovie's electrocoagulation device has hardly changed in almost a century. It has been refined and made safer, and the circumstances in which it is used have to comply with much stricter requirements than in the pioneering age of Cushing. However, although the whole concept of electrocoagulation can now be considered completely safe, the charge administered to patients is still not much different from that generated by an electric eel – several hundred volts.

Epilogue

The Surgeon of the Future: A Top 10

ANY OPTIMIST TRYING to imagine what kinds of weird and wonderful things surgeons might be capable of in the future actually pinpoints the shortcomings of surgeons today. Science fiction has been in existence as a literary genre for more than two hundred years and, in that time, writers have often tried to imagine what a doctor or surgeon would be able to do in a time of unlimited possibilities. Sometimes their portrayals have displayed surprising insight, at others they have been ridiculously naive. Below is a top 10 of surgeons from the classics of science fiction.

10. Victor Frankenstein

Frankenstein was the ultimate do-it-yourself surgeon with an insane ambition. In Mary Shelley's 1818 novel, the mad doctor cobbles together a new being from pieces of dead bodies and uses science to bring it to life. To his great alarm, his patient proves to be an intelligent being with its own opinions. Victor becomes a slave to the monster's will, which costs him his health, his marriage and ultimately his life.

The surgeon–patient relationship has changed a lot in the past fifty years, but fortunately not with the negative consequences that Victor Frankenstein faced. Communication between patient and surgeon has increased in both directions. In the twentieth century, patients still tended to allow themselves to be led to the operating room like docile sheep, without a clear explanation of what was wrong with them or what the surgeon was going to do. If they were suffering from cancer, that was often not said in as many words, and if there were several options for treating their illness, it was frequently left to the specialist to decide which course of action would be taken, without any discussion.

Fortunately, patients became more vocal, organised themselves into support groups, and demanded more insight into the results of surgery. A modern patient will inundate the surgeon with questions before agreeing to an operation. And quite rightly. Of course that can sometimes be difficult for the surgeon but, even though a patient's opinions or demands may at times push a doctor's self-control to the limit, they will never be so bad that they cost him his health, his marriage or his life. On the other hand, surgeons also cover their backs much more these days by explaining as much as possible about the illness and the treatment. That may of course be daunting for the patient, who is not always pleased to be presented with a whole list of possible risks, complications and side effects, but it has become a fixed feature of the modern doctor–patient relationship. The downside of this improved communication is that modern patients no longer trust their doctors as in the past. They seek a second opinion more frequently, which leads to 'medical shopping' and overconsumption of health services.

9. Miles Bennell

Dr Miles Bennell was a man who told the truth but was not taken seriously. In Jack Finney's *The Body Snatchers* (1954), Bennell's patients turn, one at a time, into extraterrestrial vegetables, but no one believes him – except, eventually, his psychiatrist.

Today, surgeons are obliged to report abnormal cases and other calamities to the health inspectorate. An inquiry has to be set up to analyse what the normal circumstances would be and how it was possible that they no longer applied in the abnormal situation. This is followed by a plan of action, with a number of points for improvement, which must be assessed after a specified period. Patients unhappy about their medical treatment or how they have been dealt with by their medical carers can lodge a complaint with the complaints official or department at the hospital. Everyone is taken seriously these days – doctors and patients – no matter how strange their complaints may seem.

8. Dr Blair

In *The Thing*, the 1982 film directed by John Carpenter, a surgeon is infected while doing his work and becomes a monster himself. An extraterrestrial being arrives at a scientific research station in the Antarctic and starts taking the place of the researchers. After each killing, Blair has to perform an autopsy on the deformed body and finally becomes infected himself (he wasn't wearing a surgical mask). He withdraws from the group and changes into The Thing.

Surgeons work with knives, needles and other sharp instruments all the time, with which they can injure themselves. The patient's bodily fluids can also splash into the surgeon's eyes or find their way into small wounds. Surgeons are therefore very concerned about avoiding infection. They wear gloves when touching anything, they have all been vaccinated against hepatitis B, and they wear surgical masks, glasses and a cap to protect themselves while operating. Despite all these precautions, diseases can be transmitted to the surgeon, perhaps through a small hole in the thin rubber gloves caused by a needle or the point of a scalpel, or a stray drop of fluid that manages to get into the eye. The patient then has to be asked for permission to be tested for HIV and hepatitis C. If the HIV test is positive, the surgeon has to take antiretroviral drugs for a month to minimise the risk of infection and only engage in safe sex to prevent further contamination. Infection with HIV and other viruses is an occupational hazard in surgery.

7. Helena Russell

Helena Russell was a doctor in the not too distant future, from the perspective of the 1970s. She was a character in the BBC series *Space: 1999*, which was aired from 1975–7. As the title suggests, the series is set in 1999. The Moon has been knocked out of its orbit around the Earth. The future looks very unpredictable for the lunar colonists of Moonbase Alpha. And their surgeon is a woman – a very futuristic choice in the 1970s.

There is nothing at all about surgery that makes it unsuitable for women. Women can deal with the physical load, the responsibility, the pace of the work and the night shifts just as well as men. And they can possess just as much technical insight. Women are not by nature less technically minded than men, and they can sometimes be much better than men in social terms. And yet, female surgeons are still very much in the minority. But, with the proportion of women surgeons increasing rapidly, that may indeed change in the not too distant future. Back in 1999, however, female surgeons were still relatively rare – no more than one in eight in the Netherlands, and in England only 3% of consultant surgeons were women.

6. Men in white suits

In Steven Spielberg's 1982 film *E. T. the Extra-Terrestrial*, anonymous doctors from a secret government organisation perform their work ruthlessly on cuddly extraterrestrial E.T. Without asking, they take over the house where the young Elliott lives and transform the living room into an operating theatre. Because they do not take the time to first listen to the patient and to Elliott and his family, they don't understand that E.T.'s only problem is that he is homesick, and they make everything a lot worse than it already was.

The frontiers of surgery are being pushed back further and further. That often raises the question whether all this progress is necessary. Mottos like 'aiming not only to achieve the most humanly possible but also the most humanly desirable', or 'not only adding years to life, but also life to years' are heard more and more in recent decades. Making a good decision whether to perform an operation or not means striking a good balance between benefits for the patient – in terms of both length and quality of life – and the risks of the procedure. Both patients and surgeons can have a say in this decision. Patients are given a treatment code based on their own wishes and the nature and prognosis of their illness. Choosing full treatment without restrictions means that everything will be done to cure the patient and save his or her life. Specific treatment limits can be agreed upon, for example, that everything should be done except resuscitation, if that should prove necessary. Opting for a complete limitation of treatment means that nothing more is done to save the patient's life, and only those steps are taken that make the end of life as comfortable as possible.

Women

Although it is almost taken for granted today that surgery is practised by both men and women, the profession has been so male-dominated in the past 200 years that it seems as if women wielding surgical knives are something new. Yet there have always been respected female surgeons. Around the year 1000, (male) surgeon Abu al-Qasim Khalaf ibn al-Abbas Al-Zahrawi, better known as Albucasis of Córdoba, wrote that women who suffered from bladder stones could best be treated by a female surgeon. Descriptions of the skills of female surgeons are also to be found in twelfth century French literature. In Italy, women were trained to be surgeons as early as the thirteenth century and in France the widow of a surgeon was even allowed to take over her late husband's practice. The more than 3,000 surgeons who graduated in Salerno in the fourteenth century included eighteen women. In the same century, the surgeon at the court of the King of England was also a woman. After the Middle Ages, however, two remarkable changes of attitude led to the almost complete disappearance of women from surgery: the witch-hunts of the sixteenth century and the prudery of the nineteenth century, which prevailed until at least 1968. In the Netherlands, the proportion of women among newly registered surgeons between 1945 and 1990 was around 3 per cent. That increased to 12 per cent between 1990 and 2000. In 2010, 25 per cent of surgeons in the country and 33 per cent of those in training were women. By 2016, 11.1% of consultant surgeons in England were female.

5. Three sleeping doctors in cryogenic hibernation

In Stanley Kubrick's 1968 film *2001: A Space Odyssey*, three doctors spend their voyage on the spacecraft Discovery One fast asleep.

They were put into cryogenic hibernation at the start of the mission and are due to be woken up when Discovery One reaches its destination, Jupiter. However, while they sleep soundly, suspecting nothing, the on-board HAL 9000 computer hijacks the ship. The 'IT department' completely takes over the tasks of the three doctors and ends their lives.

Somewhere in the period of the Internet bubble, in the mid-1990s, a definite start was made on computerising health-care. Surgeons, too, had to go with the flow and accept these developments. Anyone who chose not to fell hopelessly behind. Handwritten medical records, prescriptions and referral letters are becoming things of the past. Every modern hospital has electronic patient records and all treatments, admissions, results and compli-cations are registered digitally. The number of medical secretaries has consequently decreased, with the result that surgeons now find themselves with much more work to do. It all sounds wonderful, the electronic letters and files, but there is no output without input. Computerisation has not been able to prevent a sharp increase in the volume of administration that surgeons and other medical specialists are expected to contend with. There is (unfortunately) as yet no question of computers completely taking over the tasks of human doctors.

4. Leonard McCoy

Leonard McCoy was the quiet ship's doctor on the USS *Enterprise* in Gene Roddenberry's original series of *Star Trek*, which was aired from 1966 to 1969. For a man of the twenty-third century, McCoy is quite old-fashioned. He wants nothing to do with the technology and ice-cold logic of his sparring partner Mr Spock. No evidence-based surgery nonsense for him, just good old rest, routine and cleanliness. His patients lie in the neat and tidy four-person sick bay, fast asleep. Under McCoy, there is no fast-track when it comes to post-operative care on the *Enterprise*.

In our minds, bed-rest is inextricably bound up with post-operative care. Who could ever have thought in the 1960s that lying in bed actually does more harm than good in the important phase of recovering after an operation? McCoy did have a small device, about the size of a smartphone, with which he could obtain a detailed diagnosis simply by moving it back and forth over the patient. His treatments, too, were futuristic, even if only because he could get every crew member who had been attacked by an alien back on his or her feet in no time, leaving no handicaps or scars. But there was nothing futuristic about his policy after administering this high-tech treatment: just as in the great hospitals of the seventeenth century, he would simply put his patients in bed and wait for them to recover.

3. The Robot Surgeon

In George Lucas's 1980 epic *Star Wars: The Empire Strikes Back*, an anonymous robot fits Luke Skywalker with a mechanical arm after the young hero loses his right hand in the war between good (The Force) and evil (The Dark Force). At the same time, Luke realises that the evil Darth Vader, who had hacked off his hand with a laser sword, is actually his father. Such a half-baked fairy tale always has to have a happy ending. As a kind of deus ex machina, the robot replaces the lost limb with a bionic hand. Although in this future, Luke Skywalker is a satisfied patient, surgeons seem to have become completely superfluous.

Breathtaking technical developments have been made in surgery in the past thirty or forty years. Increasingly complex operations have become possible, with smaller and smaller incisions. Remarkably enough, robotics have not played a particularly important role in that rapid progress. Certain abdominal operations can be performed using a robot, but the robot cannot be pre-programmed; a surgeon always has to control it in real time. Moreover, robotic surgery offers no new options: the same procedures can be performed without robots. Other technologies, however, such as those relating to navigation and virtual reality, are more interesting in terms of improving operating procedures. In that respect, films like *The Matrix* (Andy and Larry Wachowski, 1999) and *Total Recall* (Paul Verhoeven, 1990) present a more realistic picture of the future of surgery than *Star Wars*.

2. Dr Ash

Ash is the doctor on board the space freighter *Nostromo* in Ridley Scott's 1979 film *Alien*. When a nightmarish alien appears on board by bursting out of the chest of one of the crew members, Dr Ash thwarts the efforts of the rest of the crew to destroy it. The crew kill him and discover that he was not human, but a mechanical android that blindly followed its pre-programmed instructions. The company operating the spaceship had given the android secret orders to search for alien life. Ash was thus a doctor who follows the instructions of his board of directors to the letter, even at the expense of his own colleagues.

Medical specialists determine the quality of their care themselves. Together with the patient, they decide what is to be done and the best way to do it. This is in the hospital's interests, but hospital boards have other interests, too. They have to pay salaries, purchase medical supplies and manage the hospital building, all without spending too much money, of course. Although the same quantity of care can sometimes be provided with less money, less well-trained staff, cheaper materials and fewer facilities can naturally have a negative impact on quality. Of all the specialists in a hospital, surgeons are perhaps most dependent on well-trained staff, good quality materials and up-to-date facilities. That also makes them the most dependent on the policy of the hospital board. They should therefore be able to keep a finger on the pulse of how that policy is made. Unfortunately, surgeons have the least time of all medical specialists to do this. Generally speaking, policy-making in health care – nationally and in individual hospitals – is in the hands of managers and non-surgical doctors, while surgeons look on from the sidelines.

1. Peter Duval

Peter Duval is the handsome surgeon on board the submarine *Proteus* in Richard Fleischer's 1966 film *Fantastic Voyage*. A prominent scientist from the Eastern bloc defects to the West, bangs his head and suffers a brain haemorrhage. Only a minimally invasive operation can remove the blood clot in his brain. And that is taken very literally in this science fiction film. Using futuristic technology, a nuclear submarine, crew and all, is reduced to the size of a red blood cell and injected into the man's neck. The sub loses its way and has to take a much more exciting route to the brain, via the heart and the inner ear. To make things worse, it proves to have been a serious error to take an internist along on the voyage. As the story evolves, it becomes clear that the internist, Dr Michaels, is a spy and is sabotaging the team's well-intentioned plans. But Michaels receives his just deserts when he is devoured by a white blood cell. Surgeon Peter Duval can then put on his tough-guy diving suit and, with the beautiful Raquel Welch at his side, start zapping the blood clot with a large laser cannon.

Only a surgeon could have written such a scenario! Unfortunately, even now, blood clots are not treated by surgeons in miniature submarines, but by medicines administered by non-surgical medical specialists. Just as minimally invasive, but not as much fun.

Minimally invasive treatment is the key concept in the surgery of the near future. Operations are becoming smaller and smaller and take much less time, so that the patient experiences less discomfort and inconvenience. Moreover, fewer operations are necessary because some illnesses can just as easily be treated with drugs or non-surgical procedures. Yet surgeons will never disappear completely, or be replaced by robots or computer technology. There will always be a need for a man or a woman with a knife to save people's lives, repair damage, remove cancer and alleviate suffering.

Acknowledgements

THE ACCOUNTS IN this book are based on true events in the lives of well-known and not-so-well-known patients, based on historical sources, interviews and media reports, biographies and what others have written about them. They are not intended as an exact and complete reproduction of historical facts, but more as an interpretation of them from a surgical perspective. They appeared in abridged form between 2009 and 2014 in the *Nederlands Tijdschrift voor Heelkunde*, the journal of the Dutch Surgical Association, edited by Victor Kammeijer.

I would like to thank Boris Liberov for the correct interpretation of the Russian source on Lenin's operation, Agatha Hielkema for her additional information on Dutch medical law, Marno Wolters and the Natura Artis Magistra Zoo in Amsterdam for the interview on the electric eel, my wife Laverne and my colleagues Maurits de Brauw, Eric Derksen, Eric van Dulken and Thomas Nagy for proposing useful ideas for subject matter, and Pleun Snel for reading the manuscript and providing constructive criticism.

Glossary

Abdomen Informally known as the belly. The Greek word *laparos* is used in surgery to refer to the abdomen, e.g. laparotomy: cutting open the abdominal cavity.

Abscess Accumulation of pus under pressure between the tissues of the body. To prevent it getting worse, a ripe abscess must be opened. This rule of thumb in surgery is expressed by the Latin aphorism '*ubi pus, ibi evacua*', 'where there is pus, evacuate it'. Cutting open an abscess and draining the pus is a surgical procedure. An accumulation of pus in an existing cavity is known as an empyema. See *Pus, Incision, Drain.*

Acute Sudden or immediate (not to be confused with urgent). Opposite of chronic, persistent, not sudden. Hyperacute means very sudden. Subacute means quickly, but not sudden.

Amputation Partial or complete removal of a limb. From the Latin word *amputare,* to prune.

Anaesthesia Medical specialisation that deals with local, regional or general anaesthesia of a patient for an operation. An anaesthetist is a medical specialist qualified to administer anaesthesia.

Anamnesis Literally 'from memory'. Asking a patient about the nature, severity, development and duration of symptoms. If a doctor finds out about a patient's symptoms from others, it is called hetero-anamnesis. Anamnesis is the first part of the examination of a patient. It is followed by a physical examination and, if necessary, supplementary tests. See *Symptom.*

Anatomy Literally 'to discover by cutting'. Description of the macroscopic structure of a living being. Deviations from the normal anatomy of the body can be caused by natural differences (anatomical variations) or by an illness or disorder (pathological anatomy).

Antisepsis, antiseptic The use of antiseptics (disinfectants) to remove bacteria from the skin, mucous membrane or a wound. The first disinfectants were wine and cognac. Carbolic acid was used later, but that was too harmful to bodily tissues. Today, chemicals containing iodine or chlorine are used. Simply washing with soap and water also disinfects to a certain extent, explaining why surgeons wash their hand so often. Not to be confused with asepsis/aseptic.

Arteriosclerosis Inflammatory disease of the arteries. The inner wall of the artery is affected by accumulations of cholesterol, causing an inflammation. That creates scar tissue in which calcium carbonate can be deposited. It eventually leads to narrowing (stenosis) of the artery, which can gradually or suddenly be completely blocked (occlusion).

Artery Blood vessel that carries blood from the heart under high pressure (blood pressure). Arteries are shown in red in anatomy books, because the oxygen-rich blood is bright red in colour. The pulmonary arteries are exceptional, because the blood they transport from the heart to the lungs is oxygen-poor.

Artificial ventilation Taking over a patient's breathing artificially. That may involve placing a mask over the mouth and nose, inserting a tube into the windpipe via the mouth or nose (intubation), or making an opening at the front of the neck to provide direct access to the windpipe (tracheotomy). Ventilation can be provided with a hand-held balloon or a mechanical ventilator. The simplest form of ventilation is by artificial (mouth-to-mouth) respiration.

Asepsis, aseptic Not to be confused with antisepsis/antiseptic. See *Sterile*.

Assistant Someone who assists. A medical assistant is a health professional who supports the work of doctors and other health professionals. During operations, the other members of the team supporting the surgeon are known as surgical assistants, and may include both surgeons and paramedical staff.

Atherosclerosis See *Arteriosclerosis*.

Autopsy Examination of a dead body. See *Obduction*.

Biopsy Removal of a piece of tissue for further testing, for example under a microscope. An excisional biopsy means removing all the affected tissue. With an incisional biopsy, only part of the affected tissue is removed, leaving the rest in place. See also *Excision*, *Incision*.

Blocked arteries See *Arteriosclerosis*.

Bloodletting Draining blood. Used until well into the nineteenth century to treat all kinds of complaints. Beneficial effects based completely on superstition. See *Fleam*.

Cachexia Severe malnutrition, emaciation.

Cancer Malignant disease whereby cells in the body isolate themselves from the normal control mechanisms and multiply and spread autonomously at the expense of the body. A cancerous tumour is invasive, i.e. it actively breaks through the barriers of the body. Cancer of the skin, mucous membrane or gland tissue are referred to as carcinoma, of the blood cells as leukaemia, and of all other tissues as sarcoma.

Cardiosurgery Heart surgery. Not to be confused with cardiology, the branch of medicine that treats heart disorders without surgery.

Chirurgeon See *Surgeon*.

Chronic Persistent, not sudden. See *Acute*.

Circulatory system The system of blood circulating through the blood vessels, under pressure (blood pressure) and driven by the heart. Shock is a failure of the circulatory system.

Circumcision Literally 'to cut around'. Full circumcision is the complete removal of the foreskin from the penis. See also *Excision*, *Incision*.

Complication Undesired (and unintentional) harmful consequence of a disease, disorder or operation. Not to be confused with a side effect, which is also an undesirable consequence of a course of treatment, but is not unexpected. Complications are inherent to a form of treatment, surgical or non-surgical, and can therefore usually not be attributed to human error. See *Morbidity*.

Conservative Treatment without surgical intervention or any other direct access to the body, for example, with drugs. See *Expectative*, *Invasive*.

Curative Treatment aimed at complete cure of a disease, even if that may reduce the quality of life. In contrast to palliative, where treatment is no longer aimed at complete recovery. See *Palliative*.

Cure To restore to health without leaving scars on the body. See *Healing*.

Diagnosis Identifying what is wrong with a patient: the nature, cause and severity of the illness.

Dislocation Displacement of a bone from a joint. Also referred to as a luxation. A fracture dislocation is a combination of a dislocation and a fracture. See *Reposition*.

Divide Cutting or burning through a structure or organ in a surgically responsible manner. An intestine can be divided using a surgical stapling machine. A blood vessel is divided by cutting through it and tying it off with a ligature. See *Ligature*.

Drain *Noun*: A tube or strip inserted through an opening in the body to allow something to drain, e.g. air from the chest cavity (thorax drain) or pus from an abscess cavity. Mostly made of rubber or silicone. A special kind of drain is a urinary catheter, which is inserted into the bladder through the urethra. *Verb*: To drain fluid, more specifically used for an incision in an abscess to allow the pus to escape. The whole surgical intervention is known as 'incision and drainage', I & D for short. Sometimes a drain is left behind in the incision or inserted through a secondary incision (counterincision) to allow any pus that is still in the abscess or may form later to escape. See *Abscess*.

Dys-, dis- Prefix meaning 'abnormal' or 'troubled'. Dysphagia means difficulty in swallowing. Dyspareunia means literally 'troubled interaction' and is used for physical problems with sexual intercourse.

Ec-, ex- Prefix meaning 'out'. A tumourectomy, for example, is the removal of a tumour. See *Excision*.

Elective Not compulsory, optional. An elective operation is a surgical procedure for which there is a reasonable alternative. That means that it can be planned and there is sufficient time to postpone it or not perform it at all if necessary.

Embolism Something carried along in the bloodstream and which can cause damage in the circulatory system. A blood clot from thrombosis in the lower leg, for example, can close off part of the lung (pulmonary embolism). The same can occur with fatty tissue from bone marrow after a fracture. Air in the carotid arteries in the neck (air embolism) during carotid surgery can cause a cerebral infarction.

Embryological Relating to the development of an organism before birth. Once an embryo is sufficiently recognisable as the animal it will become, it is known as a foetus.

End–of–life care Stopping all treatment to combat a fatal disease and aiming to bring the patient's life to an end as comfortably as possible. See *Palliative*.

Enema Rinsing the bowels via the anus. Despite their widespread and enthusiastic application to alleviate a broad variety of ailments, both in the past and today, there is very little evidence that enemas are effective and their excessive use can cause side effects, which may be minor but can also be more serious.

Evidence-based Making decisions and acting on the basis of results published in the medical literature. In contrast to 'expert opinion', deciding and acting on the basis of what an alleged expert in the area concerned would do or not do. Evidence can have varying degrees of reliability. The greater the total number of patients from which a certain conclusion can be drawn, the more reliable the evidence. Evidence can lead to national guidelines to provide a framework for those providing treatment.

Excision Cutting out. Removing something in full by cutting it away completely. See also *Incision, Circumcision, Biopsy, Resection*.

Expectative Watchful waiting, not (yet) giving treatment and monitoring the patient closely. See *Conservative, Invasive*.

Exposure Freeing (if necessary by dissection) a structure or abnormal tissues, including their immediate surroundings, to give a clear view of the surgical field, including the whole structure and how it is related to those around it.

Fast track Form of post-operative care aimed at restoring the patient's normal functions as soon as possible. This includes eating and drinking, getting out of bed and walking around, and removing tubes and catheters.

Fistula Two small wounds connected to each other by a tunnel through the body's tissues. It can link one cavity to another, or a cavity and the outside world. An anal fistula, for example, connects a wound in the rectum to another in the skin. Latin for tube, pipe or flute.

Fleam Special knife used for bloodletting by, for example, making an incision in the fold of the elbow. The special form of the blade is designed to ensure that the cut does not go too deep. See *Bloodletting*.

Fluctuation Effect whereby pressing one side of a swelling filled with fluid causes it to be pushed outwards on the other side. As this does not occur with a swelling filled with solid material, checking for fluctuation will clarify whether the swelling is liquid or solid. A mature abscess, for example, will be liquid, while a swelling without an abscess will be solid. See *Pus, Incision, Drain*.

Fracture Broken bone.

Gangrene Dying off of living tissue, such as the skin around a wound, a toe or a whole limb. The dead (part of a) limb can dry out and shrivel up. That leads to black mummification and, in the best scenario, to rejection by the body. The dead tissues can also rot and discharge fluid and pus that can enter the bloodstream. Wet gangrene is therefore more dangerous than dry. Gangrene can be caused by the obstruction of an artery or by a wound infected with aggressive bacteria. Some bacteria produce gas, exacerbating the spread of the gangrene. This is known as gas gangrene.

Gout Inflammatory disease caused by an accumulation of uric acid crystals in the joints. A typical symptom is a painful, inflamed big toe. The term 'gout' was formerly used for any painful complaint of unknown cause.

Gynaecologist Medical specialist concerned with obstetrics and the surgical treatment of the female reproductive organs.

Haematuria Blood in the urine.

Healing Healing and curing are two forms of 'making people better' but, unlike curing, healing leaves its marks on the body in the form of scars. See *Cure, Surgeon, Surgery*.

Hemi– Prefix for half, used mainly to indicate a right or left half. Hemiparesis means half-paralysed, on the right or left side of the body. A hemicolectomy is the surgical removal (–ectomy) of half (hemi-) of the large intestine (colon). Not to be confused with the prefix haema- or haemo-, relating to blood.

Hernia Rupture in tissue that should normally provide strength, with the consequence that something else protrudes through the hernia. A crack in one of the intervertebral discs in the spine can cause a hernia in the neck or back, while a rupture of the abdominal wall can lead to an abdominal hernia.

Homeopathy Form of quackery, like bloodletting. See *Bloodletting*.

Idiopathic Without a clearly identifiable cause. Not to be confused with '*e causa ignota*' (e.c.i.), Latin for 'of unknown cause'.

Ileus Stagnation of the passage of the contents of the intestines through the small intestine. Causes vomiting and a swollen abdomen. A mechanical ileus, obstruction of the small intestine, is caused by a constriction, a tumour or a blockage from the inside, such as a hairball. A paralytic ileus occurs when the natural movement of the bowels (peristalsis) stops, causing the contents of the intestines to come to a halt. Ileus is not to be confused with colon obstruction, which interrupts the flow of faeces through the large intestine.

Incidence Figure indicating how often a certain disease occurs in a specific population group, mostly expressed as the number of new cases per 100,000 per year. Not to be confused with prevalence. See *Prevalence*.

Incision Literally 'cut into'. The simple action of making a cut with a scalpel. An incision into the abdominal cavity is also known as a section, as in caesarean section. See also *Excision, Circumcision, Biopsy, Drain*.

Incontinence Not being able to retain faeces or urine.

Indication In surgery, a reason to perform an operation.

Infarction Mortification of all or part of an organ as a result of an obstruction in an artery (or a branch of an artery) that supplies it with oxygen-rich blood. An infarction in part of the brain is known as a stroke. An infarction in all or part of a limb is called gangrene. See *Ischaemia*.

Infection See *Inflammation*.

Inflammation A reaction in the body's tissues characterised by the activation of inflammatory cells and pain, redness, swelling, heat and loss of function in the affected area. An infection is an inflammation caused by a virus or another living pathogen, such as a bacterium, yeast, fungus or parasite. Most infections provoke an inflammation, but not all inflammations are caused by an infection.

Intermittent claudication Oxygen deprivation in the muscles of the lower leg when walking, due to narrowing of the arteries supplying blood to the legs; and which causes pain that stops immediately during rest. See *Ischaemia*.

Invasive Treatment involving direct entry into the body via an operation or with a catheter, as with percutaneous coronary intervention (PCI). In contrast to treating an illness with drugs or by other non-invasive means. Minimally invasive treatment aims to minimise the disadvantages of an operation. See *Expectative*, *Conservative*.

Ischaemia Shortage of oxygen in all or part of an organ or limb caused by insufficient supply of oxygen-rich blood, for example due to narrowing of an artery. Symptoms include pain and loss of function, which occur or worsen as the organ or limb is used more intensively, as this increases the demand for oxygen. Extreme ischaemia leads to an irreversible infarction and the mortification of tissues. See *Intermittent Claudication*.

Laparotomy Opening the abdomen with an incision. Compare with laparoscopy, keyhole surgery in the abdomen. See *-tomy*, *Abdomen*.

Learning curve Decreasing probability of complications and death of a patient (morbidity and mortality) as a surgeon, a team or a hospital gain greater experience with a specific operation. Eventually, the risk of morbidity and mortality decreases to such an extent that gaining further experience no longer has an effect. The learning curve is then 'completed' or 'achieved'. A typical learning curve requires more than a hundred patients to complete.

Ligature Tying off a bleeding blood vessel with a thread. There is a fixed procedure for placing a ligature. The surgeon first fixes a clamp to the bleeding wound. When the bleeding has stopped completely, an assistant passes a thread behind the tissue below the clamp and ties a knot in it. This calls for communication. The assistant says 'yes' when he is finished, after which the surgeon carefully opens the clamp. The assistant then says 'thank you' if the knot seems to have the bleeding under control, after which the surgeon removes the clamp completely and gives it back to the scrub nurse. The scrub nurse then gives the surgeon a pair of scissors, which he uses to cut off the ends of the thread.

Lithotomy position Lying on the back with both legs in the air. Provides a clear view of the perineum. Preferred position for operations on the anus, vagina, scrotum and penis. Since Louis XIV, also the preferred position for giving birth.

Lithotomy Surgical removal of a stone from the bladder (literally, stone-cutting). Those who performed the operation were formerly referred to as stone-cutters.

Local Used for a location in the body that does not belong anatomically to a described region, for example, the forehead, the little finger, the navel or the pancreas. See *Regional*.

Luxation Dislocation. See *Dislocation, Reposition*.

Lymph Tissue fluid. Clear fluid between the cells transported by the blood. Special small lymph vessels remove excess lymph fluid separately. Lymph fluid from the small intestine, known as chyle, also contains fats from food, giving it a milky colour. See *Lymph nodes*.

Lymph nodes Nodes no larger than half a centimetre, where lymph vessels come together. In groups they form lymph stations on the large network of lymph vessels in the body. See *Lymph, Metastasis, Radical*.

Macroscopic Visible to the naked eye, in contrast to microscopic, meaning too small to be seen with the naked eye.

Medical error See *Complication*.

Mesentery Attachment with which the small intestine is connected to the back of the abdominal cavity over its whole length and through which blood vessels run to and from the intestine. It is shaped like a fan, so that on the intestine side, it is six metres long, but only 30 centimetres where it is attached to the abdominal wall. It is also about 30 centimetres across from the point of connection at the back of the abdominal cavity to the intestine. That is long enough to allow the intestine to protrude from the abdomen onto the operating table when the abdominal cavity is cut open.

Metastasis Literally 'displacement'. Occurs when cancer cells break loose from a tumour and form a new tumour elsewhere in the body. The metastasis can be direct, across the edges of a cavity or plane, or via the blood vessels to a more remote part of the body, for example, via the portal vein to the liver, via arteries to the bones or the brain, or via the lymph vessels to the lymph nodes.

Morbidity From the Latin word *morbus*, meaning disease. Used in surgery to describe the occurrence of complications. Can be expressed in the percentage chance that a specific complication will occur in the case of a certain procedure. See *Complication*.

Mortality Risk of death, from the Latin word *mors*, meaning death. In surgery death resulting from a disease or a surgical operation. Can be expressed as a percentage chance that a patient will die from a certain disease or procedure.

Narcosis See *Anaesthesia*.

Necrosis Dead tissue. Cutting away dead tissue is called necrotectomy.

Needle holder Surgical instrument used to hold the stitching needle firmly and guide it through the tissues.

Nervous system Collective name for the brain, the spine and the nerves.

Obduction Autopsy.

Obesity Excessive body weight that poses a health risk, compared with others of the same gender and race, and of the same age and height. Adults in the Western world are considered to be obese if their body mass index (BMI: weight in kilograms/square of their length in metres) is higher than 25. The BMI obesity limit for Asians, for example, is lower.

Occlusion Blockage of an intestine, a blood vessel, or any other hollow structure. A blocked artery can cause an infarction or gangrene. See *Arteriosclerosis*.

Operative report Documented record of a surgical procedure in a patient's medical file. A report has to be made of every operation, describing the procedure from A to Z, from the position of the patient on the operating table and the disinfecting of the skin to the final stitch and the application of the dressing. The report should also note the names of the patient, the operating surgeon, the assistant and the anaesthetist, plus the date, indication and nature of the operation.

Orthopaedics Orthopaedic surgery. Literally 'straightening a child'. Orthopaedics was originally a discipline that focused on fitting children with braces, splints, shoe inserts and orthopaedic footwear to correct deformities of the bones. Although this did not involve surgical procedures, orthopaedics has now become a specialised 'cutting' discipline, with operations being performed on the musculoskeletal structure of the body. The main activity of orthopaedic surgeons is currently replacing joints with prostheses.

Outcome (of care) The total results obtained by a doctor, team or care institution in treating a specific illness, including the negative consequences, such as morbidity and mortality, in both the short and longer term. A commonly used measure of outcome is the five year survival rate, i.e. the percentage of patients that are still alive five years after the operation.

Palliative Reducing pain without curing the cause. Palliative care is treatment aimed both at prolonging the life of terminally ill patients and improving their quality of life, but without the prospect of a complete cure. Compare with curative treatment. See *End-of-life care, Curative*.

Pathological Deviating from the normal, healthy situation. Pathology means 'the study of illness', but is also used to describe the department of a laboratory or hospital that conducts microscopic examination of tissues and autopsies.

Per primam In the first instance. Healing *per primam* is primary wound healing. See *Wound healing*.

Per secundam In the second instance. Healing *per secundam* is secondary wound healing. See *Wound healing*.

Perianal Around the anus, in the vicinity of the anus or related to the anus.

Perineum Literally the area around the opening through which we are born. The area between buttocks and the lower abdomen. Includes the pelvic floor, with the anus, vagina, scrotum and penis.

Peritoneum The inner lining of the abdominal cavity. An infection of the peritoneum is known as peritonitis.

pH value Chemical expression of the acidity of a liquid: pH7 is neutral, lower is more acidic, and higher is more alkaline. The optimal pH of the human body is 7.4.

Post-natal After giving birth. A post-natal depression is a psychological disorder, a form of depression, suffered by women after they have given birth.

Prevalence The number of cases of a certain disease in a population group at a given moment. Prevalence is mostly expressed as patients per thousand. See *Incidence*.

Primary See *Per primam*.

Primum non nocere Basic principle of medicine, meaning literally 'first do no harm'. At least, do not make a situation worse than it already is. A surgeon sometimes has to make a situation worse, by performing an operation, to ultimately improve it. In such cases, the long-term advantages and disadvantages must be considered. A decision on whether to perform a surgical procedure cannot therefore always be made on the basis of *primum non nocere*. Surgeons could better work according to the principle of 'do unto others as you would have them do to you'.

Probe Rod-shaped instrument used to probe the depth of a wound or fistula.

Prognosis Prospect. How an illness will end, the chances that it will end well or badly, the time required for recovery, the symptoms or complications that can be expected.

Prosthesis Temporary or permanent replacement of part of the body by something artificial, for example an artificial leg, false teeth, an artificial blood vessel, artificial ossicles in the ear, an artificial hip or shoulder.

Purgative A laxative to provoke diarrhoea, such as castor oil.

Pus Liquid produced by an infection, comprising dead inflammatory cells (white blood cells), bacteria, tissue and tissue fluid. Different pathogens cause different kinds of pus, with a characteristic smell, colour and texture. A typical subcutaneous abscess (boil) contains creamy, light yellow pus with a slightly cheesy smell. An abscess around the anus will smell strongly of faeces. Teeth abscesses have the most unpleasant smell. See *Abscess*, *Drain*.

Radical Literally 'roots and all'. Always used in surgery in combination with a resection or excision. Means that not only an organ or part of an organ are removed, but also the accompanying lymph nodes. Radical resection is also known as extirpation, which has the same literal meaning. See *Total, Metastasis, Lymph nodes*.

Regional Relating to a region of the body, i.e. which has its own artery and vein carrying blood to and from the organism. Examples are the upper abdomen, the neck or the lower leg. See *Local*.

Reposition Surgical action in the case of a dislocated fracture, involving pulling or pushing the fractured bones back into place. A dislocated joint can also be repositioned. A dislocated shoulder can be repositioned using Hippocrates's method (placing a foot in the armpit and pulling on the extended arm) or the Kocher manoeuvre. See *Dislocation*.

Resection Literally 'cut away' or 'take away'. In practice, comparable to excision (cutting out).

Resuscitate, resuscitation Literally means 'revive' or 'restore to life'. All the actions required to keep a victim or patient alive in an emergency.

Risk factor A situation that causes a risk of an illness or complication occurring. Malnutrition, obesity, diabetes and smoking, for example, are four important risk factors for bad wound healing.

Scalpel Surgical knife. Formerly a one-piece knife, with blade and handle joined together. Almost completely replaced in modern surgery by a separate handle into which disposable blades can be clicked. See *Fleam*.

Scar See *Wound, Wound healing, Healing*.

Scrotum Sac containing the testicles.

Secondary See *Per secundam*.

Shock See *Circulatory system*.

Side effect See *Complication*.

Sign See *Symptom*.

Sinus A cavity with an opening to the outside. In contrast to a fistula, which joins two openings.

Stenosis Stricture of a bowel, blood vessel or any other hollow structure. Stenosis of an artery leads to symptoms during physical activity. See *Arteriosclerosis*.

Sterile 1. Not able to produce offspring. 2. Completely free of any pathogens, also known as aseptic. Not to be confused with antiseptic. Surgical instruments, operation jackets and gloves are sterilised with gamma rays or hot steam under high pressure.

Stoma Opening, mouth. Mostly used for an exit from the intestines on the skin of the abdomen. A better name is *anus praeternaturalis*, literally 'beyond-natural anus'. A stoma from the small intestine is known as an ileostomy or jejunostomy, and from the large intestine as a colostomy.

Stroke Loss of function of part of the brain due to haemorrhaging or a cerebral infarction. The official medical term is cerebrovascular accident (CVA). See *Infarction*.

Subcutaneous tissue Also known as the subcutis or hypodermis. The layer of fat and connective tissues immediately below the skin. Obesity in females is typified by an increase in the thickness of this subcutaneous layer (in men, obesity is typified by the accumulation of mainly fat in the fatty tissues in the abdomen around the intestines). Superficial blood vessels, sensory nerves and lymph vessels run through the subcutaneous layer.

Surgeon Literally 'hand-worker', also chirurgeon (archaic). Medical specialist qualified to treat patients by performing operations. Restricts himself to diseases and disorders that can be treated surgically. Surgical specialisations are known as the 'cutting' disciplines.

Surgery 'Hand-work', from the Greek words *kheir* (hand) and *ergon* (work). Also the art of healing. Historically, strictly separated from medicine, which restricts itself to curing diseases without using the hands. In modern medicine, surgeons are of course also physicians and non-cutting doctors also use their hands. The difference between curing and healing, however, maintains the difference between the two approaches (cutting and non-cutting). See *Healing*.

Symptom A change in the body's normal functions noticed by a patient. A doctor cannot thus observe symptoms, but can only be told about them by the patient. Asking about the nature, seriousness and development of the symptoms is the first stage in the doctor's examination of the patient. This stage is known as anamnesis. Any abnormalities that the doctor observes or invokes in the patient are known not as symptoms but as signs. Identifying signs is the second stage and is known as the physical or clinical examination.

Syn- or sym- Prefix meaning 'together' or 'at the same time'. Symposium means literally 'drinking together'. Syndrome is the continual coincidence of different abnormalities and illnesses.

Syphilis Sexually transmitted chronic infection. Caused by the bacteria *Treponema pallidum*. Causes tissue destruction, for example, in the face, and eventually of the central nervous system. This wasting disease was ubiquitous in the nineteenth century and could not be effectively treated until after the Second World War with antibiotics.

Thoracotomy Cutting open the thoracic (chest) cavity. Another procedure for accessing the thoracic cavity is thoracoscopy, keyhole surgery in the chest. See *-tomy*, *Thorax*.

Thorax Chest. See *Thoracotomy*.

Thrombosis Formation of a clot in a blood vessel. Thrombosis in a vein (venous thrombosis) leads to accumulation of tissue fluid, which is obstructed from flowing away. Thrombosis in an artery can lead to gangrene or an infarction.

Tissue A group of cells that all have the same function. Individual tissues have specific structures, functions and properties and usually have their own blood vessels to supply them with oxygen and nutrients. A body part usually consists of different kinds of tissue, such as skin, subcutaneous tissue, connective tissue, muscle tissue, nerve tissue, gland tissue, bone and cartilage.

-tomy The suffix *-tomy* means 'cut'. A laparotomy entails cutting open the abdomen, a thoracotomy the chest (thorax) and a craniotomy the head (cranium). The suffix *-ectomy* means 'cut out'. A tumourectomy is the cutting out of a tumour. A parathyroidectomy is removal of a parathyroid gland. Try saying that ten times in quick succession!

Total Complete. In surgery, this means including the outermost margins. See *Radical*.

Tourniquet A band tied tightly around a limb. If the pressure it creates is higher than the blood pressure, all bleeding from the limb will be stopped. If the pressure is low, the blood will be dammed up in the limb and the tourniquet can be used to facilitate the tapping of blood from a vein. See *Bloodletting*.

Transplantation Transfer of tissues by detaching them completely from the body. See *Transposition*.

Transposition Surgical method of transferring tissues without completely detaching them. See *Transplantation*.

Trauma Injury or wound (from ancient Greek) caused by an external impact. This is always taken literally in surgery. A car crash, a fall, a blow, a bullet, a knife or a punch are all examples of trauma. Traumatic thus means 'causing an injury or wound'. Surgical tweezers have small pointed ends designed to grip the tissue firmly without bruising or crushing it, and are consequently called 'atraumatic tweezers'. Traumatology is the branch of surgery concerned with wounds caused by trauma.

Triad Fixed combination of three symptoms or signs that can predict a certain diagnosis. The triad for a bad surgeon, for example, is firstly blaming complications on circumstances and not on his own (lack of) talent, secondly giving his own experience priority over scientific evidence, and thirdly, not showing respect for his operating team.

Tumour Literally a growth or a swelling. Can in theory refer to any swelling, but is in practice now only used for abnormal tissue growth. This can be benign (non-cancerous) or malignant (cancerous). A tumourectomy is the removal of a tumour. See *Cancer, Resection, Excision, Total, Radical*.

Urinary catheter See *Drain*.

Urologist Medical specialist concerned with the surgery of the kidneys, the urinary tracts, the bladder and the male genitals.

Vein Blood vessel that transports blood to the heart. The adjective is venous. In anatomy books, veins are depicted in blue. The oxygen-poor blood is a dark-red colour, which has a blue tint when seen through the thin wall of a vein. Veins have venous valves, to stop the blood from flowing back downwards. Pulmonary veins are special blood vessels that also transport blood to the heart but, because this blood comes from the lungs, it is oxygen-rich. The portal vein carries blood from the intestines to the liver, not the heart.

White blood cells Leucocytes – collective name for different cells that can be active in the blood and outside the blood vessels, where they can move to any tissue of the body.

Wound Open breach of a barrier in the body. An opening in the skin is usually referred to simply as a wound; an opening in mucous membrane is referred to as an ulcer. A wound has edges and a wound bed. The healing of a wound depends on the presence of bacteria in the wound, the amount of dead tissue, the supply of blood to the edges of the wound and the wound bed, and the patient's nutritional condition. A healed wound leaves a scar, as extra connective tissue is required to bridge the opening.

Wound healing The recovery of a wound, leaving a scar. Primary wound healing is bridging the wound opening with connective tissue. It can only occur if the wound is clean, the edges of the wound are sufficiently pressed together for several days, and there is an adequate supply of blood to the wound bed and the edges of the wound. In the case of secondary wound healing, the wound initially remains open and will gradually fill up with new tissue known as granulating tissue. The skin or the mucous membrane will then close over this new tissue. See *Wound*.

X-ray image intensifier Fluoroscopy. Method that uses X-ray imaging to show fractures live on a monitor. The X-ray machine can be used during an operation. Those present in the operating room will then have to wear lead jackets to protect themselves from the radiation.

Bibliography

General Publications

Altman, Lawrence K., 'Doctors Call Pope Out of Danger; Disclose Details of Medical Care', supplement to the *New York Times*, 24 May 1981

Conan Doyle, Arthur, *Sherlock Holmes's Greatest Cases* (Crime Masterworks) London: Orion, 2002

Dekker, Pauline, and de Kanter, Wanda, *Nederland Stopt! Met Roken*, Amsterdam: Uitgeverij Thoeris. www.nederlandstopt.nu, 2008

Ellis, Harold, *Operations that Made History*, Cambridge: Cambridge University Press, 1996

Farley, David, *An Irreverent Curiosity: In Search of the Church's Strangest Relic in Italy's Oddest Town*, New York: Gotham Books, 2009

Hartog, J., *History of Sint Maarten and Saint Martin*, Philipsburg, NA: Sint Maarten Jaycees, 1981

Haslip, Joan, *The Lonely Empress: Elizabeth of Austria*, London: Phoenix Press, 2000

Herodotus, *The Histories* (ed. John M. Marincola, trans. Aubrey de Sélincourt), London: Penguin Classics, 2003

Hibbert, Christopher, *Queen Victoria: A Personal History*, London: HarperCollins, 2000

Cento Anni di Chirurgia: Storia e Cronache della Chirurgia Italiana nel XX Secolo. Eugenio Santoro, Edizioni Scientifiche Romane, 2000

Lifton, David S., *Best Evidence: Disguise and Deception in the Assassination of John F. Kennedy*, New York: Macmillan, 1980

Matyszak, Philip, *Ancient Rome on Five Denarii a Day: A Guide to Sightseeing,*

Shopping and Survival in the City of the Caesars, London: Thames & Hudson, 2007

Men Who Killed Kennedy, The, History Channel, A&E Television Networks, 1988

Mulder, Mimi, and de Jong, Ella, *Vrouwen in de heelkunde: Een cultuurhistorische beschouwing*, Overveen/Alphen a/d Rijn: Uitgeverij Belvedere/ Medidact, 2002

Norwich, John Julius, *The Popes: A History*, Chatto & Windus, 2011

Nuland, Sherwin B., *Doctors: The Biography of Medicine*, Amsterdam: Uitgeverij Anthos, 1997

Pahlavi, Farah Diba, *An Enduring Love: My Life with the Shah – A Memoir*, New York: Miramax, 2004

Pipes, Richard, *The Unknown Lenin: From the Secret Archives*, New Haven/ London: Yale University Press, 1996

Report of the President's Commission on the Assassination of President John F. Kennedy, Washington, DC: United States Government Printing Office, 1964

Santoro, Eugenio, and Ragno, Luciano, *Cento anni di chirurgia: Storia e cronache della chirurgia Das Wiener Endoskopie Museum: Schriften der Internationalen Nitze-Leiter-Forschungsgesellschaft für Endoskopie*, vols 1 and 3, Vienna: Literas Universitätsverlag GmbH, 2002

Scott, R. H. F., *Jean-Baptiste Lully*, London: Peter Owen, 1973

Sedgwick, Romney (ed.), *Lord Hervey's Memoirs*, London: William Kimber and Co., 1952

Service, Robert, *Lenin: A Biography*, Cambridge, MA: Belknap Press, 2000

Szulc, Tad, *Pope John Paul II: The Biography*, London: Simon & Schuster, 1995

Tanner, Henry, 'Pope's Operation is Called Successful', supplement to *The New York Times*, 6 August 1981

Tulp, Nicolaes, *De drie boecken der medicijnsche aenmerkingen. In 't Latijn beschreven. Met koopere platen. Tot Amstelredam, voor Jacob Benjamyn, boeck-verkooper op de hoeck van de Raem-steegh achter d'Appelmarck*, 1650

Tulpii, Nicolai, *Observationes medicae. Editio Nova, Libro quarto auctior et sparsim multis in locis emendatior*, Amsterdam: apud Danielem Elsevirium, 1672

Tumarkin, Nina, *Lenin Lives! The Lenin Cult in Soviet Russia*, Cambridge, MA: Harvard University Press, 1997

Vospominaniya o Vladimire Il'iche Lenine, vols 1–8, Moscow, 1989–91

Wilkinson, Richard, *Louis XIV*, Abingdon/New York: Taylor & Francis, 2007

Worsley, Lucy, *Courtiers: The Secret History of the Georgian Court*, London: Faber & Faber, 2010

Medical Publications

Aucoin, M. W., and Wassersug, R. J., 'The Sexuality and Social Performance of Androgen-Deprived (Castrated) Men Throughout History: Implications for Modern Day Cancer Patients', *Social Science & Medicine*, December 2006, 63(12): 3162–73

Beecher, H. K., 'The Powerful Placebo', *Journal of the American Medical Association*, 1955

Bergqvist, D., 'Historical Aspects on Aneurysmal Disease', *Scandinavian Journal of Surgery*, 97, 2008: 90–9

Bernstein, J., and Quach, T. A., 'Perspective on the Study of Moseley et al.: Questioning the Value of Arthroscopic Knee Surgery for Osteoarthritis', *Cleveland Clinic Journal of Medicine*, May 2003, 70(5): 401, 405–6, 408–10

Bretlau, P., Thomsen, J., Tos, M., and Johnsen, N. J., 'Placebo Effect in Surgery for Ménière's Disease: A Three-Year Follow-Up Study of Patients in a Double Blind Placebo Controlled Study on Endolymphatic Sac Shunt Surgery', *American Journal of Otolaryngology*, October 1984, 5(6): 558–61

Brewster, D. C., et al., 'Guidelines for the Treatment of Abdominal Aortic Aneurysms: Report of a Subcommittee of the Joint Council of the American Association for Vascular Surgery and Society for Vascular Surgery', *Journal of Vascular Surgery*, 2003, 37(5): 1106–17

Chandler, J. J., 'The Einstein Sign: The Clinical Picture of Acute Cholecystitis Caused by Ruptured Abdominal Aortic Aneurysm', *New England Journal of Medicine*, 7 June 1984, 310(23): 1538

Cohen, J. R., and Graver, L. M., 'The Ruptured Abdominal Aortic Aneurysm of Albert Einstein', *Surgery, Gynecology & Obstetrics*, May 1990, 170(5): 455–8

Dudukgian, H., and Abcarian, H., 'Why Do We Have So Much Trouble Treating Anal Fistula?', *World Journal of Gastroenterology*, 28 July 2011, 17(28): 3292–6

Eastcott, H. H. G., Pickering, G. W., and Rob, C. G., 'Reconstruction of Internal Carotid Artery in a Patient with Intermittent Attacks of Hemiplegia', *Lancet*, 1954, 2: 994–6

Francis, A. G., 'On a Romano-British Castration Clamp Used in the Rights of Cybele', *Proceedings of the Royal Society of Medicine*, 1926, 19 (Section of the History of Medicine): 95–110

García Sabrido, J. L., and Polo Melero, J. R., 'E = mc2/4 Men and an Aneurysm', *Cirugía Española*, March 2006, 79(3): 149–53

George Androutsos, G., '*Le phimosis de Louis xvi (1754–1793) aurait-il été à l'origine de ses difficultés sexuelles et de sa fécondité retardée?*', *Progres en Urologie*, 2002, vol. 12: 132–7

Gilbert, S. F., and Zevit, Z., 'Congenital Human Baculum Deficiency: The Generative Bone of Genesis 2:21–23', *American Journal of Medical Genetics*, 1 July 2001, 101(3): 284–5

Halsted, W. S., 'Practical Comments on the Use and Abuse of Cocaine', *New York Medical Journal*, 1885, 42: 294–5

Hee, R. van, 'History of Inguinal Hernia Repair', Institute of the History of Medicine and Natural Sciences, University of Antwerp, Belgium, *Jurnalul de Chirurgie*, 2011, 7(3): 301–19

Hjort Jakobsen, D., Sonne, E., Basse, L., Bisgaard, T., and Kehlet, H., 'Convalescence After Colonic Resection With Fast-Track Versus Conventional Care', *Scandinavian Journal of Surgery*, 2004, 93(1): 24–8

Horstmanshoff, H. F. J., and Schlesinger, F. G., 'De Alexandrijnse anatomie: Een wetenschappelijke revolutie?', Leiden University, *Tijdschrift voor Geschiedenis*, 1991, 104: 2–14

Kahn A., 'Regaining Lost Youth: The Controversial and Colorful Beginnings of Hormone Replacement Therapy in Aging', *Journals of Gerontology Series A: Biological Sciences and Medical Sciences*, 2005, 60(2): 142–7

Lascaratos, J., and Kostakopoulos, A., 'Operations on Hermaphrodites and Castration in Byzantine Times (324–1453 AD), *Urologia internationalis*, 1997, 58(4): 232–5

Lerner, V., Finkelstein, Y., and Witztum, E., 'The Enigma of Lenin's (1870–1924) Malady', *European Journal of Neurology*, June 2004; 11(6): 371–6

Lichtenstein, I. L., and Shulman, A. G., 'Ambulatory Outpatient Hernia Surgery. Including a New Concept, Introducing Tension-Free Repair', *International Journal of Surgery*, January–March 1986, 71(1): 1–4

McKenzie Wallenborn, W., 'George Washington's Terminal Illness: A Modern Medical Analysis of the Last Illness and Death of George Washington', *The Papers of George Washington*, 1999

Mattox, K. L., Whisennand, H. H., Espada, R., and Beall Jr, A. C., 'Management of Acute Combined Injuries to the Aorta and Inferior Vena Cava', *American Journal of Surgery*, December 1975, 130(6): 720–4

Moseley, J. B., O'Malley, K., Peterson, N. J., et al., 'A Controlled Trial of Arthroscopic Surgery for Osteoarthritis of the Knee', *New England Journal of Medicine*, 2002, 347: 87–8

Pinchot, S., Chen, H., and Sippel, R., 'Incisions and Exposure of the Neck for Thyroidectomy and Parathyroidectomy', *Operative Techniques in General Surgery*, June 2008, 10(2): 63–76

Riches, Eric, 'The History of Lithotomy and Lithotrity', *Annals of the Royal College of Surgeons of England*, 1968, 43(4): 185–99

Spriggs, E. A., 'The Illnesses and Death of Robert Walpole', *Medical History*, October 1982, 26(4): 421–8

Vadakan, V., 'A Physician Looks at the Death of Washington', *Early America Review*, winter/spring 2005, 4(1)

Voorhees, J. R., et al., 'Battling blood loss in neurosurgery: Harvey Cushing's embrace of electrosurgery', *Journal of Neurosurgery*, April 2005, 102(4): 745–52

Wilson, J. D., and Roehrborn, C., 'Long-Term Consequences of Castration in Men: Lessons From the Skoptzy and the Eunuchs of the Chinese and Ottoman Courts', *Journal of Clinical Endocrinology and Metabolism*, December 1999, 84(12): 4324–31

Index

alveoli 191

amnesia: anaesthesia 103; brain damage 31

amputation: definition 310; etymology 310; legs 110, 114–16; speed 101–2, 262; toes 140, 145

Amsterdam 17

an-: meaning 94

anaemia: blood loss 52; stomach cancer 63

anaesthesia: in brain surgery 296; definition 310; development 100–1, 102, 104–6; electric eel 288–9; local 105–6, 229, 271; modern 106–7; respiration 34

anaesthesiology 102–3

anaesthetists 73

anal fistula 8–9, 61–2, 276–9, 280–2, 284–5

analgesics 103

anamnesis 126, 310

anarchism 55

anatomy: abdomen 154, 216, 224, 226–7, 237, 238, 241; definition 310–11; terminology 201–2, 221

androids 306

aneurysms 161, 162–5, 174, 195

angioplasty 87, 256

animals 286–7

ankles 75–6, 77–8

anorexia nervosa 48

antibiotics 248

antibodies 147

antisepsis 106, 116, 311

anus 88, 276–81

AO Foundation 79

aorta 160–1, 162–4, 238

aortic aneurysm 174, 195

aortic dissection 130–1, 138

apnoea 59, 60–1, 94

appendectomy 97–8, 173

appendicitis 74, 93, 94–9, 124, 125, 195, 270

appendix 205, 286

Apronius, Lucius (junior) 150, 151, 156–7

Apronius, Lucius (senior) 150–1

Arderne, John 282–3, 284

Aristotle 125

Arms: subclavian steal syndrome 256

arteries: aneurysms 161; blockage 209, 256; blood pressure sensors 51; circle of Willis 256, 260; circulation 86, 238; definition 311; diabetes type 2 188; evolution 89; lungs 191; tobacco 189; vascular surgery 129–31; vasodilation 46

arteriosclerosis: age of patient 274; definition 311; evolution 89; modern growth in 4–5; pathology 194, 256, 259, 311

burns 47
buttocks 283–4
Byzantines 179, 180–1

cachexia 63, 312
Caesianus, Lucius Apronius 150,
    151, 156–7
callus 80–1
Cambyses, King 80
cameras 173; *see also* laparoscopy
cancer: bacteria 264; barriers
    144; colon 73; definition 312;
    development course 209;
    electric eel 290; melanoma
    145–6; metastasis 146–8, 268,
    319; modern growth in 4–5;
    non-Hodgkin lymphoma
    131–2, 136; pancreas 290;
    prostate 185–6; stages 148–9;
    stomach 62–3, 263–4, 268;
    surgery 51; terminology 94;
    tobacco 188, 189–90, 192,
    195–6; treatment 147–8, 149;
    see also tumours
carbolic acid 116
carbon dioxide 212
carcinoma 94, 312
cardiac arrest 194
cardiac surgery 51, 53–4, 189
cardiac tamponade 50, 52
cardiogenic shock 46–7, 51, 52
cardiologists 122, 174
cardiology: definition 312

cardiosurgery: definition 312
cardiovascular diseases 189
Caroline, Queen of England 3,
    209–11, 212, 213–18
carotid artery 253, 259–60, 286
Carpenter, John 300
Carrel, Alexis 129, 272
Carrico, Charles James 24, 26,
    32
Carter, Jimmy 132
cartilage 246–7
Castiglione, Giancarlo 70–1
castration 175, 177–81, 182–6,
    262
Cathedral of St John, 's-
    Hertogenbosch, Netherlands
    198
Cato 152
cause 120–1
cauterisation 292
CCD chip 173
Celestine IV, Pope 57
Çelik, Oral 65
cell membranes 144
cellophane 163–4, 166
cellulitis 143
Celsus, Aulus Cornelius 19–20,
    40, 85
cerebrovascular accident (CVA)
    see stroke
Charlemagne 41
Chauliac, Guy de 226
chemotherapy 148

childbirth 100, 104, 106, 110,
271, 273–4
chimney sweeps 189
chimpanzees 11
China 177, 178, 179
chirurgeons: etymology 1;
sixteenth century 4; *see also*
surgeons
chloroform 103, 104, 106
cholecystectomy 132, 173, 174
cholecystitis 159
cholera 107
cholesterol 59
chondrocytes 247
Christianity 39; *see also* popes
Christie, Agatha 121–2, 123
chronic: definition 312
cigarettes 187–8, 189–90, 192,
195–6
circulating assistant 73
circulation: ABC of emergency
medicine 29
circulatory system: components
46; definition 312; lungs 191,
192–3; metastasis 148; process
86–7; shock 46–7; *see also*
arteries; heart; veins
circumcision 35, 36–7, 38–41,
44–5, 291–2, 312
clamps 113, 249, 270
Clark, William Kemp 27–8
cleft palates 181–2
Clement XII, Pope 56

Clostridium perfringens 110–11,
112, 113–14
co-morbidities 235
coagulation 293; *see also* electrocoagulation
cocaine 105–6, 271
coccyx 283–4
codes of practice 18, 76, 82
colon: cancer 73; obstruction
209
colostomy 70
Columbus, Christopher 108
coma 32
complaints 300
complications 10, 234–6, 312; *see
also* morbidity
computerisation 304
conductors (musical) 139–40
Connally, John 30, 34
consciousness: anaesthesia 103;
shock 46, 50
consent 234
constipation 88
contagion 107
contour operation 157
contraception 58
corpses: dissection and hand-
washing 106; exhumed for
trial 57
corsets 53
cosmetic surgery 157
coughing blood 94
CPR 54

genic shock 46–7, 51; ECG
287; fibrillation 240; function
52, 86–7; pacemakers 57;
transplants 272; valve replacement 174; whales 287; *see also*
cardiac surgery
heart attack 194
heart transplants 130
heartburn 161
Heliogabalus 180
Heller, Thérèse 263, 265–6, 268
hemi-: meaning 315–16
Henchcliffe, Margaret 26
hepatitis 300, 301
hepatosplenomegaly 132
Heraclitus 208
hernia: definition 316; diaphragmatic 225; etymology 225;
evolutionary cause 88;
femoral 225; groin 224–5,
226–9, 230–1, 271; keyhole
surgery 168; placebo operations 205; spinal discs 225;
umbilical 3, 212–18, 219, 225
Herodotus 75, 77, 79–80
Herophilus 155
Hervey, John 214, 217
Hesiod 177
Hill, John 189
Hill, Rose 65
hip, artificial 74, 88, 270
Hippocrates 18, 22, 82, 85, 152,
281–2

Hippocratic oath 18
HIV 300
Hivites 36–7, 39
Holmes, Sherlock 126–8
holy relics 41
homeopathy 197, 198, 316
homosexuality: Lully, Jean-
Baptiste 140–1; Pope Leo X
61–2
horror carnis 62, 63
hospital policies 306–7
Houdini, Harry 10–11, 91–3,
94–5, 96, 98–9
House, William 200
hula hoops 228
Hültl, Hümér 269
Humes, James 25, 26, 29
humours 120
hygiene: bladder stones 16–17;
clean underwear 22, 142;
development 5, 11, 106;
phimosis 35–6
hypertension 235
hypospadias 182
hypothalamus 137
hypovolemic shock 47, 50
hysterectomies 172

I & D *see* drain (verb)
idiopathic: definition 199, 316
ileostomy 70
ileus 120, 209, 218, 316
Illouz, Yves-Gerard 157

Stuyvesant, Peter 11, 109–10, 111, 113, 114, 116–17
subclavian steal syndrome 256
subcutaneous tissue 323
suffocation *see* asphyxia
surgeon–patient relationship 298–9
surgeons: administrative tasks 304; attitude required 8–9; clothing 5–6, 72, 101–2, 105; competence 82; cowboys 263, 270; definition 323; diagnosis 119, 124, 127–8; etymology 1, 323; gender balance 301, 303; guilds 4; learning curve 8–9; as part of the treatment 7–8, 119, 129; Pope John XXI 58; specialisms 50–1; triad for bad 325; *see also* codes of practice
surgery: basic actions 182–3; definition 323; discovery of basic procedures 2; double-blind trials 201, 202; evidence-based 160; jargon 10; minimal invasive 173–4, 308; *mors in tabula* 236; placebo operations 205–7; planes 183; specialisms 50–1; telesurgery 168–9, 174; treatment options 208–9; *see also* emergency treatment; laparoscopy; operations

surgical instruments 112–13, 138, 204, 249, 262, 270, 271–2, 291–2
surgical technologist 73
survival rates 160, 164
suturing: abdominal wound healing 266–7; absorption 250; fish 289; knots 165; ligature communication 317–18; needles and threads 290–1; nomenclature 188; process overview 290
swallowing 62, 63
sym-: meaning 324
sympathetic nervous system 49, 51–2
symptoms: definition 323–4; diagnosis 126; waiting cure 208
syn-: meaning 324
syphilis 243, 244, 248, 254, 258, 324
Sztáray de Sztára et Nagymihály, Irma 48

Tague, James 31
Talmud 151–2, 155
tamponade 50
Taylor, Elizabeth 157
technology 242, 291, 292–4, 305–6
teeth 66, 275–6
telesurgery 168–9, 174

underwear 22, 142
Uranus 175, 176
Urban VII, Pope 57
urethra 17, 19, 22, 176, 182, 184
urgency surgery *see* emergency treatment
urgency (urination) 18–19
urinary catheter *see* drain
urination 18–19, 184
urine: bacteria 16, 17; blood 94; shock 46
urologists 51, 325
Usher, Francis 228–9
uterine fibroids 172
uvula 205

Van der Heijden, Luc 168, 174
van Savoyen, Carel 22
varicose veins 3, 84, 85–6, 87–8, 205, 279–80
vascular prosthesis 163, 166
vascular surgery 51, 87, 129–30, 189
vasoconstriction 46, 47, 52
vasodilation 46
veins: bloodletting 204; circulation 86, 237; definition 325; intravenous drip 264; portal 87; valves 83–4, 86; varicose 3, 84, 85–6, 87–8, 205, 279–80; vascular surgery 129–30
Vercelli 62

vertebrae 88
vertigo 199
Vesalius, Andreas 221, 227
vestibular system 199, 200
vets 286
Victoria 100, 102, 103–5, 107
virtual reality 306
viruses: cytomegalovirus (CMV) 71; fever 137; infection 38
vision, brain damage 31
vitallium 249
vocal cords 182
Volkmann, Richard von 105
vomiting of blood 63
votive offerings 198

waiting 208–9
Waldenström's macroglobulin-aemia 136
walking 4
walking upright 84–5, 88–9
Walpole, Robert 219–20
war 109; *see also* battlefield wounds
Warren, Earl 26
Warren, John 101
Warren Commission 26, 30, 236
Washington, George 32–3
Weisz, Bess 99